Praise for
THE PRICE OF PANIC

"Jay Richards, William Briggs, and Douglas Axe have written the definitive account of the most egregious policy blunder in the history of American government."
—George Gilder, author of *Life after Google*

"As America emerges from lockdown, many are wondering how we were all stampeded into actions that have caused more deaths than they prevented. How did 'experts' like Fauci become gods, and why were those of us who questioned the panic labeled as 'psychopaths'? How did progressive fascism become the 'new normal' and, more importantly, how do we get—and keep—the normal normal back? Arm yourself with the answers to these questions by reading *The Price of Panic*, then buy a copy for a liberty-minded friend."
—Steven W. Mosher, author of *Bully of Asia: Why China's Dream Is the New Threat to World Order*

"We physicians appropriately focus on an individual patient's medical problems as we see them before us; very few of us have the knowledge or wisdom to balance the much larger issues involved in responding to public health pandemics with major economic and political impacts. This book puts these issues in perspective, for example, by showing that the illness and death toll from the COVID-19 virus was unremarkable in comparison with many historical pandemics. 'What was remarkable is how we reacted' is how the authors put it. They explore this and other important issues, such as why the COVID-19 pandemic incited worldwide panic whereas previous pandemics did not. This book also shows how most decision-makers relied way too heavily on gimmicks, such as computer models, to arrive at disastrous decisions. As a radiologist, I saw how my X-ray film seemed like magic to others; I had to resist the temptation to imply that I actually had magical powers to tell other doctors what to do."

—Robert J. Čihák, M.D., past president, Association of American Physicians and Surgeons

"Practically everything the Internet told you about COVID-19 is wrong. While the pandemic may have been real, the panic was more a product of social contagion. Jay Richards, William Briggs, and Douglas Axe provide a highly informed, page-turning look at how the entire world succumbed to what can only be described as a virus of experts."

—Austin Ruse, author of *Fake Science: Exposing the Left's Skewed Statistics, Fuzzy Facts, and Dodgy Data*

"Entertaining prose, surprising insight, and an engrossing account of how a handful of so-called experts with bad track records, dubious modeling, and no data convinced world leaders to shut down the economy. This book exposes the 'expert-media industrial complex' and confirms the lesson that 'nothing spreads like fear.'"

—Betsy McCaughey, Ph.D., *New York Post* columnist

THE PRICE OF PANIC

THE PRICE OF PANIC

HOW THE TYRANNY OF EXPERTS TURNED A PANDEMIC INTO A CATASTROPHE

DOUGLAS AXE
WILLIAM M. BRIGGS
JAY W. RICHARDS

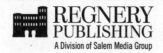

REGNERY PUBLISHING
A Division of Salem Media Group

Regnery® is a registered trademark of Salem Communications Holding
Corporation

ISBN: 978-1-68451-141-9
eISBN: 978-1-68451-142-6

Library of Congress Catalog Number: 2020939344

Published in the United States by
Regnery Publishing
A Division of Salem Media Group
300 New Jersey Ave NW
Washington, DC 20001
www.Regnery.com

Manufactured in the United States of America

10 9 8 7 6 5 4 3 2 1

Books are available in quantity for promotional or premium use.
For information on discounts and terms, please visit our website:
www.Regnery.com.

From Douglas Axe

To Daniel and Emily, who, like countless other young people, had their big day taken away, and to Verna, who, at ninety-one, refused to let fear steal a day.

From William M. Briggs

To my dad, who taught me to be skeptical of experts.

From Jay W. Richards

To my daughters, Gillian and Ellie, who survived being trapped in the house with me while this book was being written.

CONTENTS

INTRODUCTION

*What can we be certain of from history? That human
beings have been wrong innumerable times, by vast
amounts, and with catastrophic results. Yet today there are
still people who think that anyone who disagrees with them
must be either bad or not know what he is talking about.*

—Thomas Sowell[1]

The last century gave us the word "viral" to refer to the spread of
tiny pathogens. It didn't take long for the meaning of the word to
expand. We now speak of stories and ideas "going viral" when they
explode into public awareness.

In 2020, the metaphor reclaimed its literal sense.

UN secretary-general Antonio Guterres declared the greatest crisis
since World War II. In the United States, state and federal governments
ordered the closure of tens of thousands of small businesses—many
never to return. Almost every school and college in the country sent its
students home to finish the school year in front of their computers.
Churches cancelled worship services, many before the government
forced them to. Christians celebrated Easter in their homes, in front of
screens. Overnight, "social distancing" went from an obscure medical
term to a duty. Shaming of skeptics on social media was ratcheted up
to ever-new heights.

A walk in the park became a criminal act. In Brighton, Colorado, police handcuffed former state trooper Matt Mooney in front of his six-year-old daughter. Why? He was playing tee-ball with her in an otherwise empty field.[2] Police cited a Pennsylvania woman "out for a drive" during stay-at-home orders.[3] Michigan governor Gretchen Whitmer banned family visits between homes. A ninety-nine-year-old man in New Jersey was charged for attending an engagement party with nine other people.[4]

This was not a top-down dictatorship imposed on a resistant public. Polls showed that most Americans supported the lockdowns. If anything, we pushed for them. Neighbors snitched on small church groups with gusto. New Jersey posted a form on its website to make it easy to turn your neighbors in to the authorities.[5] In late March, Los Angeles mayor Eric Garcetti said that "snitches" in his city would "get rewards."[6] Two months in, most Americans were still telling pollsters that they supported the shutdowns.

Local government did its best to keep up. On Easter morning, District of Columbia mayor Muriel Bowser tweeted that she had met with the Easter Bunny. "It expressed its frustration about people not staying home," she reported, "and consequently, that its stops may be delayed this year. We agreed that road closures will be necessary for the Easter Bunny to quickly hop its way through the District and stay on time."[7]

Louisville mayor Greg Fischer tried to ban drive-in church services on Easter. A federal judge quickly slapped that down.

In the Philippines, President Duterte ordered police and the military to shoot residents who wandered out.[8] Thank God we live in the land of the free.

All this in response to a new virus—a tiny infectious agent that hijacks living cells.

Some viruses are deadly, and the coronavirus that causes COVID-19 certainly can be. Symptoms of the disease may include fever, coughing, shortness of breath, chest pain, and loss of smell. Severe cases can lead to pneumonia, and even death. More than four hundred thousand deaths worldwide by the end of June have been attributed to the virus since we first detected it at the end of 2019. By the end of May, it had claimed about a hundred thousand souls in the United States. At its peak, on Good Friday, April 10, just over two thousand Americans were reported to have died with it in a single day. There were later apparent peaks. But these followed the Centers for Disease Control (CDC) diluting the way COVID-19 deaths were coded, which increased their numbers.

Death is always hard, and these numbers sound shocking. Context matters, though. When we compare COVID-19 deaths to the background death rate and to deaths in other pandemics, the situation looks different. This virus triggered global panic long before it compared to any other global catastrophe. As we'll show in these pages, even after several months, total U.S. deaths were well below those of several twentieth-century flu pandemics. None of these triggered a global panic, and some are now almost forgotten. The global response to COVID-19 vastly exceeded that to any other pandemic in history. The president of the Philippines issued his shoot-to-kill order before his country of over 100 million people had suffered 150 deaths.

Never before had scores of countries around the world chosen to perform such economic harakiri in unison. In the United States, unemployment was at a historic low of 3.5 percent in February. By the week ending May 2, 33.5 million new jobless claims had been filed over a mere seven-week period. There had never been anything like this in American history. Ever. By the end of May, the new jobless claims had climbed to nearly 41 million.

This was not a bottom-up panic, as in the movie *Contagion*, where people need no inducement to fear a deadly virus that melts skin and dissolves organs. Sure, people bought more toilet paper, as they do when forecasters predict severe weather. They also snapped up hand sanitizer. But there were no riots and little civil unrest during the first month, even when cases and deaths were going up. Our panic led, at first, to compliance and self-protection.

So, what caused the viral panic? The panic and lurching government overreach were inspired not so much by deaths people knew about firsthand, and not so much by the virus's murky origins in China. They were sparked by a few forecasts that had the smell of science. The World Health Organization (WHO) favored a single, untested, apocalyptic model from Imperial College London. The United States government took its cues from the Institute for Health Metrics & Evaluation (IHME) at the University of Washington. We now know these models were so wrong they were like shots in the dark. After a few months, even the press admitted as much. But by then vast damage had been done.

How powerful were these false prophets? In describing his choice to wage war on the invisible enemy, President Trump told the press on April 8, "The big projection being that 2.2 million people would die if we did nothing. That was another decision we made, close it up. That was a big decision that we made. Two very smart people walked into my office and said listen these are your alternatives. And that was a projection of 1.5 to 2.2 million people would die if we didn't close it up."[9]

"Two very smart people." Let that hang in the air for a minute.

As we soon learned, the IHME often had to adjust its forecasts to align them with the facts.[10] These weren't random errors. Their tweaks always went in one direction: fewer deaths, fewer needed hospital beds, and so forth, than they had forecast the day before.

By April 10, Anthony Fauci, M.D., the president's top medical advisor and surely one of those "two very smart people," was insisting that he didn't follow models.[11] Never mind that twelve days before, he had brandished models to dissuade the president from loosening the reins at Easter. "We showed him the data," Fauci explained, "he looked at the data, and he got it right away. It was a pretty clear picture."[12]

On April 11, the IHME tweeted, "We strongly agree that decision-makers should draw on a diversity of COVID-19 models. We're committed to scientific debate and constant improvement of our predictions."[13] Model defenders cited the much lower rates of deaths as proof—not that the models were wrong, but that the shutdown had worked.[14]

As we'll see, that's not true. Whether we compare countries or U.S. states, the virus seemed indifferent to government-mandated lockdowns. Not only did the models exaggerate the danger, but our response to that danger, both voluntary and coerced, exacted great pain for little or no gain. That may sound baffling. How could a nationwide shutdown not stop or at least greatly slow a contagious virus? But as we'll see, there is no evidence it did.

Add to this the spectacle of the CDC changing the way that it (and the U.S.) counted COVID-19 infections and deaths, which caused a spike in the death count in mid-April. At that point, it was not just the models, but also the underlying data that were iffy. It was as if our public health officials were trying to spark conspiracy theories.

It's easy to grasp why the public, and even heads of state and other politicians, trusted public health experts in a perceived public health emergency.[15] But what of those experts? They treated predictive models—which are at best complex conjectures about future events—as if they were data. And then, when the models flopped, they began to massage the data. To get past this catastrophe we will need to forgive, but we should never forget. We should do whatever we can to dismantle such experts' unchecked power over public policy.

These experts, however, could never have done so much damage without a gullible, self-righteous, and weaponized media that spread their projections far and wide. The press carpet-bombed the world with stories about impending shortages of hospital beds, ventilators, and emergency room capacity. They served up apocalyptic clickbait by the hour and the ton.

For the U.S. media, facts and nuance took a back seat not just to hysteria, but also to bloodlust against the president. The anti-Trump angle persisted even as the narrative about the virus changed. In January the press attacked Trump for restricting travel from China against advice from WHO. They called it a xenophobic reaction to a virus that wasn't passed from person to person. Later, the press blasted the president for not clamping down sooner. As a result of this spectacle, millions of Americans knew they couldn't trust the press to give them the straight scoop. And the president knew that, no matter what he did, the press would attack him for killing people.

Without media hype, we doubt the panic over this virus would have gone viral, or that most governments would have responded as they did. As it was, only a few managed to resist the tide of misinformation across the globe—Taiwan, South Korea, Singapore, Sweden, Japan, Hong Kong, and a few others. And in the United States, only Iowa, Oklahoma, Nebraska, North Dakota, South Dakota, Arkansas, Utah, and Wyoming didn't have lockdowns, though many of their counties and cities did.

Social media made COVID-19 the first virus "with public relations,"[16] as an Israeli physician and former health minister put it. We were incessantly fed secondhand tweets of people sick or dying, liked and retweeted thousands of times. Any effort to quell fear by, say, comparing the outbreak with past pandemics, disputing the models, or urging a more targeted quarantine was denounced as tantamount to murder.

On April 4, an open-air fish market at the Wharf in Washington, D.C., drew a crowd of shoppers. City police soon closed it, egged on by an army of online scolds who took to Twitter to denounce the fish-seeking sociopaths as soon as the story broke and for twenty-four hours afterwards. There were scores of such incidents in cities around the country.

Every celebrity who tested positive, from Tom Hanks and P!nk to Idris Elba and Chris Cuomo, found his or her way to the front page. UK prime minister Boris Johnson garnered the most attention. But even the fifty-two-year-old guy from Fountains of Wayne who died with the virus trended for a few days.

Of course, people, even famous ones, get sick every minute of every day. One hundred and fifty thousand people you've never heard of die every day somewhere in the world. Starting in March, though, the ever-relentless media made juicy stories look like evidence. Coverage of the virus was so pervasive that some obituaries of those who died at that time noted that the deceased *hadn't* died of COVID-19. No stories noted that people had not died of heart disease or cancer—though they killed far more people over those same months.

We were hooked on news analyses with eye-catching graphs. Millions spoke, like statisticians, of "flattening the curve." We mistook rumors of millions of deaths and emergency rooms overflowing with bodies for reports when they were dubious worst-case scenarios. Major media outlets went so far as to use deceptive pictures of busy hospital wards captured at other times and places. News stations ran with memes that were too good to check, like the absurd viral video of a nurse who "quit" her ICU nursing job because her hospital wouldn't let her wear a mask. It wasn't true, but CBS reported it, and Senator Bernie Sanders fell for it.[17]

Of course, we were all affected by the virus in some way. Many of us got sick or knew someone who did.

Between us, we three co-authors know several people who landed in the hospital. One of us has a friend whose father died in Bergamo—the ground zero of the pandemic in Italy.[18] You have your own stories.

But our experiences don't prove that a plague was shrouding the earth in darkness and death via a pandemic of such magnitude that no response was too extreme. The press spoke in terms of a war economy as firms shifted manufacturing from cars (GM), pillows (My Pillow), and vodka (Tito's) to ventilators, masks, and hand sanitizer.[19] But our fear of the coronavirus did what no real war, depression, terror attack, or disease had ever done before. It not only emptied hotels and airplanes. It shuttered professional baseball and basketball and the Summer Olympics. It closed schools, businesses, and churches. It kept healthy people with near-zero risk of death huddled in their homes for months.

They say hindsight is 20/20. But here we are, months later, and most of us still have more questions than answers. How much did social distancing, school and business closures, stay-at-home orders, and press campaigns help? What will be the total cost in dollars, lives, and livelihoods of this response from governments and mass media? What role have national and global health organizations such as WHO played? To whom are they accountable? How did unelected bureaucrats with narrow expertise, relying on murky data and speculative models, gain the power to shut down the world?

And why did elected politicians, who knew little of the science, trust them?

How much of the blame belongs to social media mavens and reporters who amplified the claims of officials? What of a TV talker who wore a hazmat suit to terrify viewers, while his unseen cameraman wore a t-shirt? Or White House correspondents who frittered away press conferences with the president, badgering him about what he called the virus? What of headlines that aimed for clicks and political digs rather than truth and accuracy?

And, amidst all this, what of average citizens? How are we supposed to sift prudence from propaganda? How can we tell when we should quietly comply rather than openly question? With the collapse of media credibility, whom should we trust if something like this happens again? Given what we saw from officials and the media, is it any surprise that so many people fell for conspiracy theories?

Was this a unique event, never to be repeated, or a harbinger of a "new normal"?

We can answer that last question now: it depends on whether we learn the right lessons this time.

Enemies of the American experiment, both inside and outside our borders, were watching. They now know that even the most liberty-loving Americans will surrender our rights if we think the lives of other people, especially the vulnerable, are at risk.

There's a book to be written about the many acts of generosity and bravery by charities and donors,[20] businesses, health care workers, servicemen and women, police, firefighters, government workers, artists, pastors, priests, and ordinary folks in the United States and around the world.[21] This is not that book.

In this book, we diagnose and dissect the response to the crisis by the public, the press, and the government. Historically, it's during crises that governments expand their reach. And unfortunately, they almost never retreat after the crisis has passed. Alas, the panic over COVID-19 has given rise to an expert-media industrial complex. It has the power to trigger public panic, which in turn inspires government overreach. These experts and their like-minded media heralds now have even more incentive to use our fear and our compassion against us.

To resist this new force, the rest of us need a way to distinguish evidence from extrapolation, and data from models. We need to know just how hard it is for scientists and physicians to tease out the many causes that contribute to death in human populations. We need to be able to tell truth from truthiness, and wisdom from hokum. To know when experts are trustworthy, and when they're blowing smoke.

We need to know what happened and how it happened, so we can keep it from happening again. Or the coronavirus will turn out to be the least of our problems.

CHAPTER 1

WHERE DID THE PANDEMIC START?

[T]he only thing we have to fear is fear itself—nameless,
unreasoning, unjustified terror which paralyzes needed
efforts to convert retreat into advance.

—*Franklin Delano Roosevelt*[1]

A hundred years from now, someone may write a book about the pandemic panic of 2020. It will have a catchy title like *Extraordinary Delusions* or *The Madness of Crowds*. It may be the last word on the subject. This book is one of the first. We wrote it while we were still in the throes of the crisis, fueled by a sense of futility, each of us more or less stranded in a different part of the world: one of us was in Taiwan, one in L.A., and one in Washington, D.C.

Why the hurry? Because "experts" were already warning that COVID-19 could make an encore performance for the 2020–21 season. We wanted to help prevent our country and the world from making the same disastrous mistake again.

The timing makes our job tough, though. Almost any historical event has many causes. It's much easier to tease them apart after some time has passed to provide critical distance. We can't hope to capture the detail and nuance that will only come with more hindsight. Still, even at the peak of the panic, the wellsprings of the catastrophe were in plain sight—more than enough to tell the basic story.

Fear Itself

Most of us know the fear of sickness or death. Infection provokes special fear because we can catch and spread a disease unawares. We've heard about nightmarish, organ-melting viruses such as Ebola, but they tend to show up in far-off places. We look to Hollywood to supply us with surrogate experiences of deadly pandemics. During the lockdown in March and April of 2020, millions of us streamed these movies on Netflix, Amazon, and Hulu: *Contagion* (2011), *Outbreak* (1985), *It Comes at Night* (2017), and *Twelve Monkeys* (1995). Even a few zombie movies are more science than supernatural, such as *28 Days Later* (2002), *28 Weeks Later* (2007), and *I Am Legend* (2007).

Stephen Soderbergh's *Contagion* hit close to home. It's about a deadly virus that jumps to humans from a bat—a fact the viewer learns only in flashback at the very end of the film. Bulldozers disturb the bat while it's eating a banana in a rainforest...in China. It finds shelter in a pig farm, where it drops a bit of banana. A pig eats the banana and gets infected. A chef in Macau slaughters the pig and serves it—and the virus—to patient zero, an American woman played by Gwyneth Paltrow. Her horrible if hasty death is the first of many.

The heroes of the story include not just her husband, played by Matt Damon, but surprisingly attractive officials at WHO and the CDC. (The producers consulted with WHO officials when writing the script.) These public-health savants quickly figure out that, if not stopped, the virus will kill a third of the global population. True to their role, they devise a vaccine and save the world, but not before a year of mayhem and death.

Such films are terrifying, of course. That's why we watch them. Who would watch a movie about hay fever? But they're fiction. What we tend to experience in the real world is mostly colds and the flu, which we take in stride. Indeed, we take the deaths of large numbers of people in stride.

We have to. Otherwise, we would all be in a full-time planet-wide panic. Over 1,700 people die of heart disease every day in the U.S. Over 1,600 die of cancer. Almost 700 die just from medical mistakes.[2]

With the coronavirus, however, our fear went viral. The ad for *Contagion* nailed it: "Nothing spreads like fear." In 2020, the world of frightening fiction seemed to infect our perception of reality, so much so that we elevated presumed COVID-19 deaths above all others. The usual ways of dying became background noise in the hysteria.

We knew early on that many people, especially children, seemed to catch the virus and develop antibodies without ever showing symptoms. For others, it triggered flu-like symptoms—weakness, fever, cough, sore throat, and the like. Some people, especially older ones in poor health, developed severe symptoms, including pressure or pain in the chest, trouble breathing, and bluish lips or face.[3] When death occurred, it came in the form of pneumonia. Symptomatic cases of COVID-19 were often more severe than a common seasonal illness. But this wasn't Ebola. Judged by its death rate and its other effects, the 2020 coronavirus was like a really bad flu strain, which targets people at higher risk of death while leaving most of the young and healthy unscathed.

The world has seen several flu strains like that in the last generation or two. The 1968 Hong Kong flu, for instance, took an estimated one million lives globally. The more recent swine flu (2009) killed between 150,000 and 600,000. (More on these later.) But in neither case was there global panic. Why, then, did we panic over this strain of coronavirus? Why did we retreat to our homes by the millions even before governments ordered shutdowns?[4] If we want to avoid a repeat of 2020, we need to find the answer.

BORN IN CHINA

The origin story didn't help. In late 2019, Chinese media began to report on a mysterious pneumonia-like illness cropping up in Wuhan, a giant city in the province of Hubei in central China (population over eleven million). The *New York Times* first mentioned the story on January 6 and reported the first death in China less than a week later. From the very start, the Chinese authorities seemed to suppress information about the virus that caused the illness. They went so far as blocking the hashtag #WuhanSARS on social media[5] and punishing brave Chinese whistleblowers.

On January 22, the *Times* reported that China was "cutting off" Wuhan. Chinese authorities were "canceling planes and trains leaving the city, and suspending buses, subways and ferries within it."[6] The sheer size and speed of the shutdown stunned the world, and the tight lips of Chinese officials only made the tension worse.

Comparisons to SARS and even Ebola started to show up in the Western media. But most reporters were still fixated on the impeachment trial of Donald Trump, which started on January 21. Three days later, President Trump first tweeted about the events unfolding in China: "China has been working very hard to contain the Coronavirus. The United States greatly appreciates their efforts and transparency. It will all work out well. In particular, on behalf of the American People, I want to thank President Xi!"[7]

On January 26, Senator Tom Cotton sent a letter to the secretary of Health and Human Services asking the White House to consider blocking travel from China. He briefed administration officials the next day, even missing several hours of the impeachment trial. Later he told the Senate that what was happening in China was "the biggest and the most important story in the world."[8]

Four days later, President Trump tweeted, "Working closely with China and others on Coronavirus outbreak. Only 5 people in U.S., all in good recovery."[9]

The president, long a harsh critic of the Chinese regime, was clearly biting his tongue. He had announced a coronavirus task force the day before. And the day after, he declared a national health emergency and began restricting travel from China, as Tom Cotton had suggested. At that time there were a mere seven reported cases in the United States, and the Senate impeachment trial was still grinding along.[10]

What happened next should come as no surprise. Trump's political and press critics accused him of xenophobia. Speaker Nancy Pelosi was urging tourists to come to San Francisco's Chinatown in late February.[11] Within weeks, though, the same critics would be complaining that Trump should have acted sooner.

In truth, Trump wanted to avoid a U.S. response to the virus that did more damage than the virus itself. Nevertheless, his skepticism about China likely inspired him to do far more to limit the spread from that country than Pelosi and other China-friendly critics would have.

In any case, the anti-Trump "heads-we-win-tails-you-lose" strategy that would govern the press coverage was already in place.

WAS THE VIRUS—OR ITS LEAK—ENGINEERED?

Beijing deserves a generous portion of blame for the spread of COVID-19. But that doesn't mean, as some have claimed, that the coronavirus was a product of Chinese bioengineering.[12]

Like computer viruses, natural viruses are coded scripts that trick information processors into running them. But with disease-causing viruses, the information processors attacked are biological *cells*. So, the virus's first trick is to gain entry to cells—something it usually does with appendages that can grab matching appendages on the target cells. Once attached, a virus particle can force itself into the cell and release its viral script. The cell then runs this script as if it were its own genetic script, slavishly producing more virus particles, which are released to infect other cells.

One documentary claims that the appendages (called "spike proteins") on the new coronavirus (SARS-CoV-2) are suspiciously like the appendages on the original SARS virus, which caused an outbreak in 2003. The claim seems to be that scientists engineered a coronavirus from bats so that it would infect humans: "The high similarity of the S proteins from SARS1 to now SARS2…that's your spike protein. That's the lock and key. That's going to be what drives it right through human cells…. So now you're allowing that access to human tissues."[13]

Like all proteins, these spike proteins are made in cells by linking amino acids to produce long chains that fold up into their working form. So, if someone made the SARS-CoV-2 spike protein by splicing pieces of the original SARS spike protein into the spike protein from a bat virus, we should see this. Specifically, when we examine the amino-acid sequence of the SARS-CoV-2 spike protein, we should see pieces that match the SARS-CoV-1 spike protein, with the rest matching the bat spike protein.

As Figure 1.1 shows, we see nothing of the sort. There are only three extended regions where the new coronavirus (SARS-CoV-2) spike protein differs from the most similar bat virus spike protein. Even in these regions, the SARS-CoV-2 protein is more like the bat virus protein than the SARS-CoV-1 spike protein. At the six key places for grabbing the appendages on human cells,[14] the SARS-CoV-2 spike protein is equally unlike the spike proteins from SARS-CoV-1 and the bat coronavirus (one

Spike protein region 1:

```
SARS-CoV-1:  TRNIDATSTGNYNYKYRY
SARS-CoV-2:  SNNLDSKVGGNYNYLYRL
   Bat CoV:  SKHIDAKEGGNFNYLYRL
```

Spike protein region 2:

```
SARS-CoV-1:  GKPCTP-PALNCYWPLNDYGFYTTTGIGYQ
SARS-CoV-2:  STPCNGVEGFNCYFPLQSYGFQPTNGVGYQ
   Bat CoV:  SKPCNGQTGLNCYYPLYRYGFYPTDGVGHQ
```

Spike protein region 3:

```
SARS-CoV-1:  L----LR
SARS-CoV-2:  NSPRRAR
   Bat CoV:  NS----R
```

Figure 1.1. Full spike protein sequences for SARS-CoV-1,[15] SARS-CoV-2[16], and bat coronavirus RaTG13[17] were aligned using Clustal Omega.[18] Amino acids are represented by conventional, 1-letter abbreviations.[19] Using position numbering for SARS-CoV-2, region 1 runs from 438 to 455; region 2 runs from 477 to 506; region 3 runs from 679 to 685. Dots indicate matching amino acids. The SARS-CoV-1 sequence is greyed except where there is a match between the two SARS sequences and a mismatch between SARS-CoV-2 and the bat coronavirus. Boxes show positions known to be important for infecting human cells.

in six matches either way). Bottom line: if someone tried to make the SARS-CoV-2 spike protein resemble the SARS-CoV-1 spike protein, they did a miserable job.

Despite the lack of evidence, theories about a human origin of the new virus floated around the internet. In June 2020, Tech Startups reported that Norwegian virologist Birger Sørensen had co-authored a peer-reviewed paper that "claimed the novel coronavirus SARS-CoV-2 is not natural in origin."[20] Not true. Rather, his paper's acceptance in *QRB Discovery* gave Sørensen the opportunity to offer his hunch about the origin of the virus to the press.[21] But his peer-reviewed paper makes no such claim.[22] It does talk about short pieces of sequence having been inserted into the spike protein, but this often happens naturally.

Given what we know, then, the safest conclusion is that the new coronavirus is of natural origin.

Be that as it may, did the Chinese authorities intend to infect humans with the virus? This also seems far-fetched. If they wanted to test it, they surely wouldn't have picked an industrial center—Wuhan is often called China's Chicago. They would have picked some obscure place in the far-flung northwest, set up controls, run the test, and buried the evidence. As things happened, the virus threw the regime into a tailspin and seriously damaged a reputation it had spent decades and billions of dollars cultivating.

So what happened? For a few months, the press and the World Health Organization went with the "Chinese wet market" story. Anyone who pointed to evidence that the coronavirus may have leaked from the Wuhan Institute of Virology was dubbed a conspiracy theorist. But the evidence kept growing and finally overcame whatever spell the media was under. We know this lab studied bats infected with coronaviruses. Two years before the outbreak, U.S. Embassy officials had warned about lax safety standards at the lab.[23] And in May 2020, NBC obtained a report from British and American intelligence which said that "there was no cellphone activity in a high-security portion of the Wuhan Institute of Virology from Oct. 7 through Oct. 24, 2019, and that there may have been a 'hazardous event' sometime between Oct. 6 and Oct. 11."[24]

At the time of writing, we can't settle these mysteries. The thought that the virus was released from a lab, whether by malice or incompetence, isn't crazy. But that isn't our interest here. The details around the bug's origin may have been suspicious. To find the seeds for global panic, though, we have to look elsewhere.

CHAPTER 2

WHO STARTED
THE PANIC?

Science is the belief in the ignorance of experts.

—*Richard Feynman*[1]

As a social contagion, the pandemic panic was global. No country escaped it. It should be no surprise, then, that a group with global reach and global aspirations played a key role.

WHO

You've heard of the World Health Organization (WHO). It's the arm of the UN that focuses on international public health. It was there at the founding of the UN. As its own ad copy says:

> WHO began when our Constitution came into force on 7 April 1948—a date we now celebrate every year as World Health Day.
>
> We are now more than 7,000 people working in 150 country offices, in six regional offices and at our headquarters in Geneva, Switzerland.[2]

During the 2020 pandemic, WHO's director-general was (and still is) Ethiopian microbiologist Tedros Adhanom Ghebreyesus, a noted expert on malaria. He is affiliated with a party in Ethiopia called the Tigrayan People's Liberation Front—a communist and ethno-nationalist party. (Tigray is both a region and an ethnic group in Ethiopia.)

Prior to becoming the head of WHO, Tedros held key political offices in his country, including minister of health. When elected to his post at WHO, one of his priorities was "universal health coverage."[3] China supported his election to the top WHO office in 2017. And from the start of his tenure, Tedros and WHO itself seemed to do the bidding of the communist regime. As Nicholas Eberstadt and Dan Blumenthal remarked in the *New York Post*, the World Health Organization appeared to be "Beijing's handmaid."[4]

Yeah, we know this sounds like something out of a self-published conspiracy novel you'd find at a gun show.[5] But we promise we're not making this up. The guy directing the global response to the coronavirus was a long-time communist who wanted socialized medicine worldwide. He was working hand-in-glove with the communist government of China, where the COVID-19 pandemic had originated under murky circumstances. There's no reason to think he was the wisest or best person to lead the effort…and some reason to think he wasn't. In April, Berkeley research scientist Xiao Qiang told *The Atlantic*: "Particularly at the beginning, it was shocking when I again and again saw WHO's [director-general], when he spoke to the press…almost directly quoting what I read on the Chinese government's statements."[6]

Kathy Gilsinan, a contributing writer to *The Atlantic*, remarked on the same disturbing phenomenon, "The most notorious example came in the form of a single tweet from the WHO account on January 14: 'Preliminary investigations conducted by the Chinese authorities have found no clear evidence of human-to-human transmission of the novel #coronavirus.' That same day the Wuhan Health Commission's public bulletin declared, 'We have not found proof for human-to-human transmission.'" In fact, the Chinese government was offering caveats not included in the WHO tweet. "The possibility of limited human-to-human transmission cannot be excluded," the bulletin said, "but the risk of sustained transmission is low."

Again, this is *The Atlantic*, which you never find at gun shows.

Gilsinan interpreted the overlap between WHO's tweet and the Chinese regime's propaganda statement charitably. She concluded that the regime had "deceived" WHO. But by mid-April, when her piece came out, everyone paying attention knew that WHO was compromised.

Back in January, when President Trump had first restricted travel from China to the United States and the mainstream media lambasted him, the director general of WHO was right there with them. The president's policy, Tedros said, would "have the effect of increasing fear and stigma, with little public health benefit." Even as WHO announced a public health emergency at the end of January, Tedros was still denying there was any reason to restrict travel to and from China. "Let me be clear," he said, "this declaration is not a vote of no confidence in China."[7]

To get the real scoop at the time, apparently you needed to be listening to conspiracy theorists at gun shows.

But in late March a crack in the façade was exposed by an interview with Canadian physician Bruce Aylward, a senior aide of Tedros. The intrepid reporter was Yvonne Tong of the Hong Kong–based news source RTHK.

In light of Taiwan's success in fighting the coronavirus, Tong, interviewing Aylward by video link, asked whether WHO would reconsider granting membership to the country. Aylward sat there, silent, twitching, for six long seconds. Tong finally said, "Hello?" Aylward then responded, "I'm sorry, I couldn't hear your question, Yvonne."

"Ok, let me repeat the question," she said.

"No, that's okay. Let's move to another one then," he replied.

Hmm. That's not what you say if you haven't heard a question. Tong didn't buy it, and she asked about Taiwan again. At that point Aylward hung up. Tong called Aylward back, but he was still evasive. When she asked him again about Taiwan's response to the virus, he insisted that "we've already talked about China." He then quickly ended the interview.

The Canadian Aylward, an official of WHO, part of the United Nations, was taking the Chinese Communists' line on Taiwan, which they deny is a separate country.

You have to see the video to believe it.[8] WHO found it so embarrassing that it stripped Aylward's English bio from its website.[9] The episode cratered respect for WHO among Americans who noticed. Add to that WHO's weird claims and backtracks on everything from hydroxychloroquine to masks. In May, a story broke saying German intelligence had concluded that Chinese leader Xi Jinping had asked WHO on January 21 to withhold data that the coronavirus could be transmitted between humans and to hold off on declaring a global pandemic.[10] If true, China was responsible for a deadly information lag of six weeks that left the rest of the world unprepared for the pandemic.

Even before that bombshell, when President Trump announced in mid-April that the United States—WHO's top donor—would stop funding the organization, his base cheered.

THE RISE OF THE EXPERTS

But by that point the damage was already done. WHO had helped China cover its tracks for several crucial weeks. And it had pushed a model from the Imperial College London that projected forty million deaths from the virus worldwide. This model—a piece of mathematical guesswork—was the source of the shocking but bogus claim that 3.4 percent of coronavirus infections were fatal. That's a good *thirty times* more deadly than the flu in a severe season. For comparison, the 2018–19 flu had a case mortality rate of about 0.1 percent. Policymakers should have been skeptical. Instead, that number became the basis for their response. With the backing of WHO, the dubious Imperial College model gained official status, as did a few experts with narrow specialties. At the time this book went to press, Google was still reporting the 3.4 percent fatality rate as settled fact.

Without WHO, then, the pandemic panic might never have gone global.

In response to the scare that WHO's actions had exacerbated, if not created, the governments of most countries and of most U.S. states mandated lockdowns. They closed schools and businesses, issued shelter-in-place rules, and imposed quarantines on healthy populations. In Spain, you couldn't leave your house. The same was true in some parts of the United States.

In mid-March, President Trump started holding nightly news conferences with members of the White House Coronavirus Task Force. That group was led by Vice President Mike Pence, one of only a few calming influences. Its coordinator, Dr. Deborah Birx, and Dr. Anthony Fauci, director of the National Institute of Allergy and Infectious Diseases, were soon household names.

At first these people, along with CDC leaders, took their cues from the Imperial College model. It was the basis for the original White House campaign "15 Days to Slow the Spread."[11] Other models then came to the fore. The most notable were those run at the Institute for Health Metrics & Evaluation (IHME) at the University of Washington. We'll say more about models later. For now, suffice it to say that when dealing with something as complex as a pandemic, such models are, at best, educated guesses—always wrong in the details, but sometimes helpful in showing what we don't know. At worst they're bundles of prejudices wrapped in pretentious academic packaging.

Alas, the coronavirus pandemic featured more of the latter than the former. No one should doubt that the main models, and government officials who trusted them, played an oversized role in creating the panic.

We don't think forecasters are stupid or evil. Nor do we think public health advisors want to harm people. The problem came when the press, public health advisors, and political leaders all accepted these models uncritically and relied on them in their reporting to the public and in their public policy decisions. These forecasts should have been treated for what they were—one-sided conjectures from people focused on a narrow part of a multi-part problem. As one commentator in the UK put it on Spiked, "This is where things have fallen apart. The experts have set the goal, and the politicians have cast themselves in the role of their spokespeople."[12] This gets things backwards. It's not the job of immunologists, epidemiologists, and other narrow experts in the bowels of the administrative state to make policy decisions. That's the job of elected leaders who are accountable to voters. It falls on them to make the tough calls that require weighing competing interests and perspectives.[13] For all their imperfections, politicians are apt to be more trustworthy than narrow experts when it comes to such choices.

Add to this problem the incentives that influence a public health official such as Anthony Fauci. For career safety, it's much better to overstate than to understate the risk. Put yourself in Dr. Fauci's place. Imagine you predict that a hundred thousand people will die but only a thousand really do. The result? Everyone will be relieved and soon forget that you overshot. But predict a thousand deaths and then get a hundred thousand? Time to find another job and hire police protection.

Anyone taking the advice of such officials should remember this incentive and discount their advice accordingly.

Yet even in mid-April, when we knew the expert forecasts were way off, the press was still treating Dr. Fauci as a prophet bringing stone tablets down from the mountain. He had already proved himself a single-minded technocrat, who thought the cost of a shutdown was a mere "inconvenience." But there he was on CNN on April 12, suggesting the president hadn't heeded his shutdown advice earlier.

"We look at it from a pure health standpoint," he said. "We make a recommendation, often the recommendation is taken, sometimes it's not."[14] A month and a half earlier, on February 29, he sang a different tune. "Right now, at this moment," he told the Today show, "there is no need to change anything that you're doing on a day by day basis."[15]

In mid-May Dr. Fauci was warning of the danger of "needless suffering" if states reopened "prematurely." He implied that the lockdown should continue until a vaccine could be developed. He neglected to mention that the FDA has never approved a vaccine for any coronavirus and allowed it to be brought to market.[16]

To be fair, Fauci mostly resisted the media's baiting to speak ill of the president.[17]

And when the facts kept changing, he finally came around. The real problem was that the press and follow-on Twitterati acted as if advice from an immunologist should trump the many factors that the president—any president—had to balance in such a crisis. They called Dr. Fauci the "nation's most trusted health expert." They never addressed the obvious question: Most trusted by whom? Their adulation of this single expert filtered down to the public, and up—to mayors, governors, and the president.

The U.S. media might have behaved more rationally if Hillary Clinton had been in the White House. With Donald Trump as president, though, the press played a pivotal role in putting the panic in pandemic.

FLATTENING THE CURVE

The number of deaths the coronavirus was predicted to cause depended on the model and date of prediction. In late 2019, a Johns Hopkins model simulating the outbreak of a generic disease—not the coronavirus itself—predicted some sixty-five million deaths. The fact that the modelers hadn't created the model with the coronavirus in mind didn't stop others from applying it. Other early models using "artificial intelligence," that is, statistical models with fancy names, said fifty-three million. Bill Gates came in with the lowest early forecast of thirty-three million. Another tech pro said forty-three million. The figure of fifty million became popular, perhaps because it was a round number.[18]

These scary numbers helped prod the public to panic. But, as we noted above, the estimate of forty million deaths from Imperial College London became the favored forecast. We'll have a closer look at the Imperial College and IHME models in chapter 7. For now let's consider how these tools, in the wrong hands, could be used to stir panic.

We all saw graphs illustrating the need to "flatten the curve." Vox produced the most viral version, which Barack Obama tweeted to his 117 million followers.[19] It looked something like this:

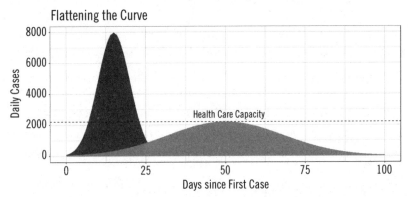

Figure 2.1. Graphs like this were used to educate the public on the meaning of "flatten the curve."

There are two curves: a high-peaked one and a flattened one. The high-peak curve represents predicted daily cases of COVID-19 without protective measures; the flat one, with protective measures. Channeling their favored experts, the media said we must avoid the high peak and aim instead for the flattened one. Why? To prevent hospitals from being overwhelmed by sick patients in the early weeks by staying below the dashed line. The idea wasn't to reduce the total number of cases, but rather to ensure proper care of the inevitable severe cases. "A flatter curve," as an article at Live Science explained, "assumes the same number of people ultimately get infected, but over a longer period of time."[20]

It's a compelling image, but it's also far too simple. We should not compress healthcare capacity into a single number. In the real world, there are ER doctors, ICU doctors, different kinds of nurses, and other personnel. There are ventilators and many other kinds of equipment. There are medical supplies of every kind. There are ER beds and ICU beds and general hospital beds, beds for general surgery and post-surgery recovery rooms. There are differences between regions. The list goes on and on. Quantifying this vast and varied collection of resources in one number is unrealistic.

We can count resources, such as ICU beds, in one hospital or in one area. But our count won't include the extra resources that would open up when people are forced to improvise. Necessity is the mother of invention. Time pressure may limit our chance to improvise, but the "flatten the curve" picture ignores it altogether.

Another problem is that the models upon which the two curves were built run on total cases. But *total* cases is the wrong thing to focus on if the concern is hospital capacity. For that we should instead focus on the fraction of cases that require treatment. Nobody had a good estimate of that when these models were being used to scare everyone in March. Only later did we realize how small this fraction was.

EMERGENCY POWERS

The chart showing the flattened curve is a reminder that in 2020, governments across the planet invoked emergency powers in the name of public health. They need these powers when there's no time for public debate. Think of bombs raining on Pearl Harbor, or airliners plunging into the twin towers and the Pentagon. But the trigger for emergency powers in 2020 was not a catastrophe that had just happened, but rather a prediction about what might happen.

The details varied from state to state. One of us co-authors (Jay Richards) lives in Maryland, which had a fairly typical response. During our lockdown, leaving home on non-essential business was a misdemeanor that could be punished with up to a five-thousand-dollar fine and one year in jail.[21]

Much of the developed world adopted similarly draconian measures. In New Zealand, even when the deaths attributed to COVID-19 were in the single digits, the government got to work issuing laws in the name of science. The result was their COVID-19 Public Health Response Bill. It stipulated that "an enforcement officer can enter, without a warrant, any land, building, ship, aircraft, or any other place or thing if they have reasonable grounds to believe that a person is failing to comply with any aspect of an order." Citizens who failed to comply faced criminal liability, with jail sentences up to six months.[22]

By the end of May 2020, most people had forgotten the curve-flattening story and most states were easing up. But the CDC still issued a sixty-page list of guidelines detailing "Activities and Initiatives Supporting the COVID-19 Response and the President's Plan for Opening America Up Again."[23]

The things we give up for safety.

CHAPTER 3

How It Spread

Until you realize how easy it is for your mind to be manip-
ulated, you remain the puppet of someone else's game.

—*Evita Ochel*[1]

Mathematical models have no power to cause panic on their own. To do real damage, they need to be taken up by power brokers and sold to the public at large. For this, the modelers need the media. Traditional media—and now social media—*mediate* between governments and the governed. A million times more people saw the media-generated curve-flattening chart than would have understood the mathematical models that inspired it.

Alas, when it comes to reporting technical details such as model predictions, the reach of the media tends to exceed their grasp. As Holman Jenkins acerbically put it in the *Wall Street Journal*, "Please, if you are a journalist reporting on these matters and can't understand 'flatten the curve' as a multivariate proposition, leave the profession. You are what economists call a 'negative marginal product' employee. Your nonparticipation would add value. Your participation subtracts it."[2]

It really comes down to how professional and social media reporters convey information they don't fully grasp. Caution would call for, first, passing things along without any preaching, and second, digging to see whether other experts may have different views. But caution is a rare commodity in a world where the main goal is to score political points or to get clicks, likes, and retweets.

How to Create a Panic, Step One: Excessive Noticing

But imagine a different scenario. How might the pandemic have played out if 1) we hadn't seen the astronomical levels of media hysteria—especially social media hysteria—that we did, and 2) experts motivated to err on the side of doomsday scenarios hadn't dominated the public response to the virus?

Picture an autumn setting. The newspaper headlines are about something a politician said. Half the country greets it with applause, the other half with outrage. Further down the front page, a celebrity speaks about a subject she knows nothing about, and a grateful nation welcomes her words.

Buried at the bottom is a small item. A person has died of an illness doctors say was likely caused by a virus.

A week later, the news is much the same. Only now, somewhere nearer the top of the page comes the report that sixteen people have died from the virus.

Another week later, with eighteen new cases, journalists are asking the sources on their contact lists why the deaths might be increasing. They report that "questions are raised about the deaths."

News of the virus's death toll now takes top spot each day. Before long, deaths have rocketed to 118. This grows to 165 in another week and 259 the week after. Experts warn of an exponential rise. Everyone gets a crash course on doubling times. Doctors warn that the virus will stress hospitals, maybe to the breaking point, unless something is done. Nobody knows what this "something" is—just that it better come quickly.

Politicians scramble. The Drudge Report posts pictures of the awful demise of some of the virus's victims. Another outlet quotes the neighbors of a man who had said, "I'm not worried about this thing" and then died of it a week later. Public mood shifts to the opinion that scoffers like that have it coming. New deaths in the United States break one hundred a day, then more than two hundred a day—*each and every day.*

Panic and fear are everywhere. In the worst week, 1,626 deaths are recorded. The news is all virus, all the time.

Then, just as politicians are ready to issue shelter-in-place orders, deaths fall to 1,179 a week, a clear decrease. The order is delayed. Predictions of a second spike, based on a computer model, go viral. The pitch of the panic is still feverish.

Yet the drop proves real. For the first time in two months, a week passes with fewer than 1,000 deaths. The next week it's down to 738. Then only 500.

"We're not out of it yet!" warn the nation's top experts. The *L.A. Times* runs a story under the headline: "Californians are losing their fear of the virus, setting the stage for disaster." But even as they broadcast their fear, the weekly deaths drop below one hundred to fifty-three. Then forty-three. Then twenty-six.

The following week we all forget the virus and return to other outrages *du jour.* Until next year, when the cycle repeats. As it would every year if we gave a blow-by-blow account of the seasonal flu in the United States.

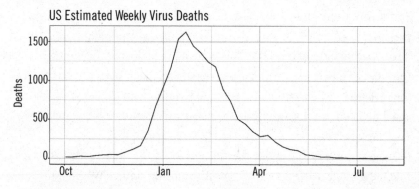

Figure 3.1. The CDC's estimated weekly flu deaths in the United States in the 2017–2018 flu season.

Apart from that *L.A. Times* headline,[3] the hype in the above account is fiction. But the death numbers are real. We have taken them from the 2017–18 flu season. The numbers change every year, but the general shape of the peak in Figure 3.1 repeats every year, not just in the United States, but throughout the world.

In the early months of 2020, the coronavirus caused a similar peak in deaths in the tens of thousands. As with most viral outbreaks, there was a slow ramp-up. Then the exponential virality—the perfect time for the press to induce tension and fear. Then the virus reaches peak morbidity and lingers for a bit, allowing the media to sustain a frenzy for a while. At some point, though, the numbers plummet, at which point the reporters ought to move on.

We aren't suggesting that the coronavirus was just like the flu. It wasn't, as we'll see later. Our point is that a blizzard of breathless reporting every hour for weeks on end could whip up a decent panic over the flu every year, if we had the stomach for it. All it would take is the earnest effort of journalists, experts, and politicians, and a skittish and gullible public, to ignite this kind of overreaction. Social contagion is as real as viral contagion, and it can be just as deadly. Imagine what would happen if they combined forces. Well, we don't need to imagine it, do we?

Social contagion—wide-scale panic—doesn't happen every year with the flu because we think of the flu as a normal part of life. We expect it and know there's not much we can do about it. We produce vaccines every year, and they do some good. Warnings to wash hands and cough into elbows might help a little. But indoor living during the winter allows the virus to pass easily from person to person. That in itself starts to slow the outbreak. More people having had the flu means fewer who can still catch it. Then, the arrival of the spring sun and outdoor living helps wash away any last remnants.

We know all this about the flu, but it's different when a new virus takes the stage with a strange, sci-fi sounding name. While mutations bring us a new version of the flu virus every season, the changes are small. On the other hand, when a virus jumps from animals to human beings, as the coronavirus did, it really is a new thing. Perhaps its novelty inspired the press to push worst-case scenarios instead of more likely ones. Sober reporting would have served the common good, but it would have driven far less traffic to news sites. We got far less truth than we needed, and far more panic.

How to Create a Panic, Step Two: Obsess over Cases

And there was another pathway to panic—fixating on "cases." Ideally, what we would like to know during a virus outbreak is how many people are infected now, and where they are. A flashing scarlet letter *I* appearing at the moment of infection would do the trick. Alas, this doesn't happen. We were well past the peak of the coronavirus outbreak by the time people began to realize that mass testing never really answers these questions.

For example, after we knew that the coronavirus had become epidemic in China and that people from the affected area had traveled to the United States, anyone could have guessed that travelers had brought the virus here.

So, how many U.S. citizens carried the virus in, say, mid-January 2020?

We don't know. It's not just that few, if any, coronavirus tests were available. It's that at first no one was checking for the virus. Why would they, before they knew about it? And you can't find what you don't test for. All manner of respiratory viruses float around all the time. There's no program to track and record every one of them. Nor should there be. And even when a virus is at its peak, it will pass over most people.

Consider Washington state, home to 7.6 million people. By the end of June, no one knew the precise coronavirus infection rates. But based on estimates, we might guess about 10 percent of the population, some 760,000 people, had been infected. The remaining 6.8 million people likely had not caught the virus.[4] It isn't unusual for a virus to pass over a large chunk of any population.[5]

Some with the virus had flu-like or pneumonia-like symptoms. Some of these people succumbed and died. Others thought they had a cold. Still more never noticed anything.

Most people who tested positive for the virus were very unlikely to be killed by it. Yet officials used these tests to inflate the COVID-19 death numbers. In Washington state, 13 percent of official COVID-19 deaths "involved persons who had previously tested positive for COVID-19 but did not have the virus listed anywhere on their death certificate as either causing or contributing to death." They were counted in the coronavirus deaths because of the "state's practice of counting every person who tests positive for COVID-19 and subsequently dies, even if the death was not caused by COVID-19."[6]

These included several deaths from gunshot wounds.[7] On top of that, healthcare workers sometimes counted people who died with coronavirus-like symptoms as dying from the coronavirus, even if they *hadn't* been tested.[8]

As testing expanded, the number of people who had tested positive (and negative) for the virus went way up, even as deaths went down. By mid-June, the press mostly reported only on "new cases" rather than deaths.[9]

If deaths were dropping across all age groups, how were "cases" rising? Well, no doubt the bug was still out there. But a parallel drop in deaths among everyone from young adults to people in their late eighties and nineties (look ahead at Figure 6.5) suggests that the virus had come close to running its course. Still, more testing meant more infections detected. Some people got tested because their employer asked them to. Others got tested while being treated for unrelated illnesses. When states were locked down, many people had avoided going to the doctor or hospital for all manner of ailments not related to the coronavirus. After the lockdowns eased and they returned to have their bunions checked, their doctors gave them routine coronavirus tests and found either an active or past infection. They had to report these. Hence the "surge" and "spike."

The press, of course, almost never distinguished new cases from old. They reported all new positive test results as if they revealed deadly new infections.

In mid-June, the press trumpeted that Oklahoma had recorded its "highest single-day increase" in cases.[10] They forgot to report that Oklahoma drug stores had just started free testing, with even more stores offering the test in the latter half of June.[11] So no one should be surprised that over half of all COVID-19 cases in the state "were recorded in the month of June."[12] Testing was also ramped up by official policy.

By the end of June, the United States as a whole was testing about half a million people *every day.*[13]

By June 27 there had been almost 2.5 million reported positive tests and 119,156 coronavirus-attributed deaths in the U.S. Taking those numbers naively implies a death rate of 4.7 percent. That's clearly false. The true case fatality rate was much lower—perhaps 80 times lower—as we know because of research using careful sampling.[14]

What happened is that most infections and cases escaped official notice, whereas no deaths did. As we noted above, most who had the bug never had treatment, and many didn't even know they had been infected.

Even death counts have built-in errors. Policies influence the numbers as much as pathology does—or even more so. We'll go into more detail in chapter 6. The basic point is that both the number of active cases and the number of deaths from the virus can be exaggerated. Not everybody who gets infected gets tested. Not everybody who tests positive has the disease. Not everybody who gets the disease dies. And not every person who dies *with* the virus dies *from* the virus. The number of infections, in contrast, tends to be greatly underestimated.

The obsession first with the fatality rate, and then with the cases, was a prescription for panic. Attention to the mean age and health of victims and comparisons to prior pandemics that hadn't provoked panics would have been much healthier medicine.

How to Create a Panic, Step Three: Compare Kiwis to Tangelos

Nobody knows how many people died of the flu last year. Or the year before that. Or any year. Nobody knows the *exact* number, that is. The best we can ever do is estimate, using a statistical model.

One paper explains the challenge of counting flu deaths:

> In non-pandemic years, influenza-associated death is mainly restricted to the elderly and people with underlying chronic illnesses. However, analyses of death certificates show that clinicians often do not attribute influenza-related deaths to influenza, but rather to a pre-existing underlying condition. [The opposite problem from what we saw in 2020, when deaths with other contributing factors were attributed to COVID-19.] Influenza-associated deaths may therefore be hidden not only among cases of pneumonia but among other causes of death such as cardiovascular events or metabolic disorders. Hence, all-cause mortality has been found to be better for assessing the total impact of the flu on mortality.[15]

Since we don't know the true tally of flu deaths, we must estimate from the fluctuations in total deaths. The idea is to plot all deaths by time, as in Figure 3.2.

It's easy to spot the yearly cycle, with deaths peaking each winter. If you look more closely, you can also see that the numbers are gradually trending upward over the years: the total population grows with time, and more people means more deaths.

To estimate flu deaths, a model is fit to this yearly cycle and to the upward trend. The result is a smooth, wave-like curve with a slight upward trend, superposed over the actual numbers. This is illustrated in Figure 3.3 with European data from EUROMOMO, which collects statistics on deaths (and deaths by age) from Austria, Belgium, Denmark, Estonia, Finland, France, Germany (Berlin), Germany (Hesse), Greece, Hungary,

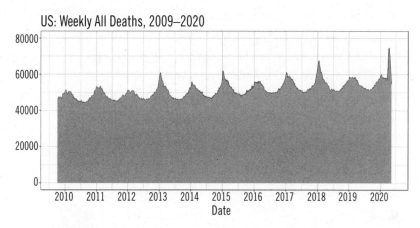

Figure 3.2. Weekly U.S. deaths by all causes (CDC). This plot is produced from three separate official CDC sources.[16] One runs from 2009 until 2019; the second begins in 2014 and continues until week twenty of 2020; and third starts at 2020 and includes COVID deaths.

Ireland, Italy, Luxembourg, Malta, Netherlands, Norway, Portugal, Spain, Sweden, Switzerland, UK (England), UK (Northern Ireland), UK (Scotland), UK (Wales). In the striped bar on the far right, instead of actual data, there is an estimate to compensate for delays in reporting.

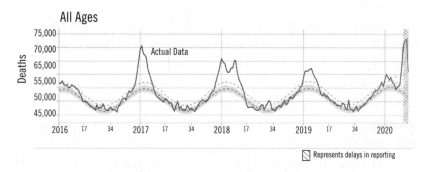

Figure 3.3. Weekly deaths by all causes in the European countries listed in the text (solid line), along with mathematical models that attempt to capture the overall trend (dashed lines).

Figure 3.3 shows two dashed lines representing two aspects of a statistical model, which you can see smooths the data. For now, don't worry about the differences between those lines. Just notice the difference between the actual data (solid line) and the smoothed trends (dashed lines). It's easy to see how the peaks each winter stick out above the waves. Those peaks sticking out above the dashed curves represent what are called "excess deaths." These excess deaths every flu season, which can be attributed to the flu, are summed for each annual flu season to get the estimated number of flu deaths for that year.

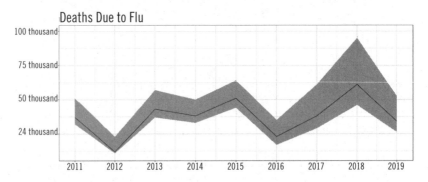

Figure 3.4. Estimated annual excess deaths by season from influenza in the U.S. (2011–2019). Years indicate year when flu season ends.

Figure 3.4 shows how the estimated flu deaths vary from year to year as a black line, with "confidence" bounds shown in gray.[17] (The number for the 2019–20 season had not been reported when this book went to press, but the CDC prediction is about twenty-four thousand deaths.)

Until recently, this complicated method for estimating flu deaths didn't receive much public scrutiny—because people usually don't panic over the flu. Before 2020, had you ever even wondered how many people died of the flu every year? Be honest.

The plot in Figure 3.4 is yearly, so it's peaky and spikey on one-year intervals. But you could also graph weekly data. That line would be much smoother over the course of a year. Alas, this difference led some otherwise serious writers to make serious blunders during the crisis. And it was inevitable that hyper-partisan, fear-mongering reporters would bungle the details.

Indeed, even the calmer, more objective media made mistakes. "Not Like the Flu, Not Like Car Crashes, Not Like…" was the title of an article written by three editors of the *New Atlantis*. You can get the gist of it from their chart for the United States (they did a similar one for New York, which has the same problems). The *New Atlantis* is a fine publication that often challenges conventional wisdom. But in this case the editors made a big mistake.

United States: Reported New Deaths Weekly

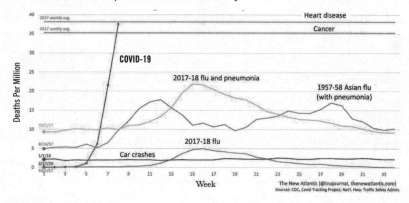

Figure 3.5.

Actual counts of reported coronavirus deaths by week are represented by the steep line labeled "COVID-19." In contrast, heart disease and cancer deaths are shown on top as estimates from averages. Car crash estimates are at the bottom, and flu estimates for some previous years are in the middle.

The *New Atlantis* editors said, "It's about the spike."[18] It sure is. But not in the way they say. No one should compare that spike with smoothed estimates, as the authors did, since it misleads.

Let's assume those coronavirus death counts are accurate (as we've seen, they're likely exaggerated). The editors were still comparing actual data (for coronavirus deaths) with smooth estimates derived from models (for the flu). And smoothed estimates from models will always make actual counts look spikey in comparison. The picture makes the corona-virus look far worse than the 1957–58 Asian flu, which is nonsense. The Asian flu killed between one and two million people that year, according to the best estimates,[19] whereas the coronavirus is winding down at a lower number—perhaps eight hundred thousand or so.[20]

It's not over, and all the studies aren't in. At this point, though, it looks like there might be about as many deaths from the coronavirus as in the 2009 swine flu, which isn't even pictured in the *New Atlantis*'s chart: between 152,000 and 575,000 dead, with a median estimate of 364,000. The 1968 Hong Kong flu isn't pictured, either. That killed an estimated one million people.

Mistakes like these mattered. They fed the press's daily breathless reporting on the coronavirus. One of us had an exchange with a well-known blogger who was passing around exaggerations and horror stories about the coronavirus on Twitter. When I pointed out that the death numbers for the Asian flu had been far worse, the gentleman was incredulous. Why, he hadn't even *heard* of Asian flu! Yet he was suggesting to his readers that the coronavirus would be our doom.

Imagine if the press had reported the Asian flu numbers non-stop for months on end. The terror that strikes our hearts would have been four times worse, at least.

The *New Atlantis* editors admitted that "comparing [coronavirus] deaths to, say, an entire year of deaths from car crashes or influenza is not meaningful."[21] Good point. Yet they relied on that very comparison to freight the "spike" with a meaning it did not have.

They were so focused on the spike that they couldn't see the bigger picture. "Amid the statistical noise is a powerful signal," they claimed. "The question is whether we choose to see it."[22]

The good thing about spikes is that they come down quickly. Heart disease and cancer, on the other hand, keep chugging along.

While you can't help but notice the daily-counts spike amidst all those smoothed estimates, that's like comparing apples to oranges—or kiwis to tangelos. The editors of the *New Atlantis* were deceived by a statistical mirage. A lot of others saw it too. But a mirage is still a mirage, no matter how many people think they see it.

At the height of the coronavirus, countless people were trying to track the precise number of deaths in real time. That's something that no one had done for a flu-like illness before, because it can't be done. The uncertainties at that level of resolution are so vast that the effort was bound to be an exercise in self-deception. Add in media hype, and it also became an exercise is mass panic.

We'll let Bill Maher have the last word. He finally got fed up with what he called the "panic porn": "Everyone knows Corona is no walk in the park. Because you literally can't walk in the park. But at some point, the daily drumbeat of depression and terror veers into panic porn. Enough with the 'life will never be the same' headlines.... Everything looks scary when you magnify it a thousand times.... Giving the proper perspective isn't a cover-up of the truth. It *is* the truth. We need the news to calm down and treat us like adults. Trump calls you fake news. Don't make him be right."[23]

CHAPTER 4

SOCIAL MANIAS AND THE CULT OF EXPERTISE

Incestuous, homogeneous fiefdoms of
self-proclaimed expertise are always rank-closing
and mutually self-defending, above all else.

—*Glenn Greenwald*[1]

We've had severe viral pandemics over the years, but this was the first pandemic of *panic*. Sure, the media are always trying to scare us, in order to bring eyes and ears to their sites and sell advertising. You may remember how they hyped mad cow disease, which was going to affect us all. It was the same story with bird flu. And global warming, (a.k.a. climate change), Ebola, the zika virus, swine flu, killer bees, killer wasps, and on and on. On May 7, 2020, *Politico* reported on "nine disasters we still aren't ready for" in a helpful story entitled "Experts Knew a Pandemic Was Coming. Here's What They're Worried About Next."[2]

Before the coronavirus, the most recent large-scale disease disaster was the swine flu of 2009, which is estimated to have killed from two hundred thousand to over half a million people. The press and politicians certainly fueled fear back then. Why didn't that create a panic? One key difference is the growth in size and power of social media. Perhaps we reached a social-contagion threshold only in the last ten years.

Crowds were just as likely to go mad in 2009 as now. We had the media, email, the internet, and blogs. But in the intervening eleven years, we grew far more connected. Apple released the iPhone on June 29, 2007. By 2009 smartphones accounted for one quarter of cell phone sales,[3] although Nielsen estimated their penetration was only 17 percent.[4] By 2018, more than four out of five Americans had a smartphone.[5] In 2020, there were 3.5 billion people on the planet with a cell phone.[6]

Two former Yahoo employees developed the message app, WhatsApp, for smartphones in 2009. Facebook acquired it in 2014, and by 2017 had 1.5 billion users worldwide.[7]

In 2009, Twitter claimed 23.5 million users.[8] By 2020, the platform had 330 million monthly and 145 million daily users, including President Donald Trump.[9] President Obama did tweet about the swine flu in 2009, but his Twitter account was essentially a generic White House account. For better or for worse, President Trump was the first president to master this social media outlet.

Instagram started in 2010, just after the swine flu pandemic. It quickly garnered 30 million users.[10] By 2020, it had 1 billion monthly and 500 million daily users.[11] Facebook had 350 million global users by the end of 2009,[12] and by 2020 this had leapt to 1.69 billion.[13] YouTube grew to more than 2 billion monthly users and 1 billion hours of content viewed daily by 2020.[14]

These are only the biggest players. We can't forget (though we'd like to) Snapchat, Weibo (China), WeChat, Line, Pinterest, TikTok, and Reddit.

In short, by 2020, billions of us were part of a real-time global conversation. The sheer size and profusion of social media, brought directly to our eyes and ears, proved intoxicating. Networks can harness the wisdom of crowds, as with traffic apps and Google searches. But they can also unleash the madness of crowds—supercharged with video streaming. In the panic over the coronavirus, we saw not just social media, but social mania.

Correct that: we were trapped *inside* a global social mania, with no way out.

WE'RE ALL EXPERTS

The mania was part chill and part thrill. Social media provides a sense of immediacy—a way to cast your opinion onto the wider world. It offers an easy dopamine rush of participatory democracy, a free platform to signal virtue and indignation every minute of every day.

Way back in February 2020, not everyone even knew what a ventilator was. Only a tiny sliver of humanity knew how to use or repair one, or had any idea of its limits and risks. A still smaller number were equipped to make them or knew about the complexities of their global supply and delivery chain.

By mid-March, though, it seemed everyone was an expert. Everybody suddenly knew just how many ventilators every ICU in every hospital needed across the country. They knew just how many patients would die without a ventilator. They could tell you to the minute how long a COVID-19 patient would have to be hooked to a ventilator—the patient's only possible hope of life.

And it wasn't just ventilators. Everybody seemed to know about hospital staffing, ICU bed use, triage procedures, and the like. Never mind that these matters are so complex that they're hard for experts who study them full time.

Not only did everyone know about these things. They took to social media to share their wisdom with the world.

In a flash, a journalist reporting on a subject he knew nothing about triggered a hundred million quotes, either approving the words as if they were A Certified Truth From On High or condemning them as if they were A Vicious Falsehood from The Father of All Lies.

In May, CNN hosted a panel on the coronavirus. One member was teenage climate activist Greta Thunberg. Clearly, fame was her only credential, but in the new world of social media celebrities, that was enough.

Twitter, Facebook, and Instagram exploded with these kinds of commentators. "Hot takes" abounded. Everybody wanted to be first to produce a take that would go viral, or at least garner likes or retweets. Every new death, rumor, and factoid was trumpeted as if it were the moon landing. Everybody knew just what the latest trend meant and what would happen next.

Many of us wanted to be part of the story, and we found social media to be the perfect insertion tool. Early in March, when fewer than forty deaths had been attributed to the coronavirus across the state of Washington, one hospital physician took to Twitter to participate in the panic. He lamented being "surrounded by death." There was just one problem: public data revealed that his hospital had had at most two COVID-19 deaths.

After one of us called him out on this, he deleted his tweet.

There were many such incidents of people "juicing" their experiences. Many were seeking to make sense of the crisis by discovering how they fit in. And some were padding their resumes, as it were, as a way of participating in the news. In doing so they were unwittingly participating in the panic that caused a great deal of harm.

In reality, most people, including most journalists, know diddly about ventilators, or epidemiological models, or complex cost-benefit analyses, or viral infections. But social media became the preferred way to fake it—including for professional journalists. Their journalism degree didn't include virology or epidemiology or statistics. But it takes no training to recognize a scary story, and that's all you need to get clicks and be lauded for your vicarious expertise. When the clickers broadcast to all their followers, even a flimsy rumor can go viral, like some kind of reputational multi-level marketing scheme.

The problem was not lack of expertise. (As you'll see, there is plenty to criticize about the misuse of actual expertise.) All of us lack expertise in most areas. Our point is that during the pandemic, social media platforms tended to dilute and distort real expertise and allow people without expertise to spread panic by assuming a spurious authority there.

Squashing Dissenters

All of this could have happened even if the social media platforms had been what they claim to be: neutral platforms for the free and open exchange of ideas, rants, and cat-fail videos. Network effects are real. In what he calls Metcalfe's Law, George Gilder has argued that the power of a network goes up as a proportion of the *square* of the number of users.[15] But on top of that, social media platforms worked overtime to boost the signals of official experts who preached panic, while at the same time purging dissenters who urged caution and calm.

If you logged onto Twitter during the crisis, you often saw ads for approved sites for COVID-19 updates. The same with Google if you searched, as we did, for topics related to the coronavirus. Instagram offered handy plugs for WHO and the CDC right at the top of your feed.

These platforms had the power to tell people where to get information. How did they know which information was best? A better question: How did they know which information was *worst*?

In mid-April, YouTube CEO Susan Wojcicki announced that the platform would remove content they deemed "problematic."[16] Specifically, they would remove anything that went against the World Health Organization as a violation of their terms of service. Wait, was this the same WHO that had tweeted on January 14 that there was no evidence of human-to-human transmission of the coronavirus—and then later had to eat crow? The organization carrying water for the communists in Beijing? Yes, that one. Wojcicki was true to her word. Her company unplugged many videos that questioned the party line, even as that line shifted.

A striking example was a video of doctors Dan Erickson and Artin Massihi. In April, they held a press conference on KERO News 23, a station in Bakersfield, California.[17] The doctors calmly discussed data from official California sources, backed up by data from their own testing practice, concluding that Californians had "a 0.03% chance of dying from COVID." They asked whether that low rate justified closing businesses and requiring the entire state to shelter in place. Their message went out to millions on Fox News, and after being posted on YouTube channels, it garnered another five million views.

YouTube answered by playing whack-a-mole—policing the platform for channels showing the video in an effort to block it. But nothing dies on the internet, so the video still shows up on the original news site and elsewhere. In a humorous twist that the officious Wojcicki didn't foresee, the purge itself made the news, raising the doctors' profiles higher than if YouTube had just stuck to their job.

Facebook's Mark Zuckerberg went on ABC news to explain why his company had tried to memory-hole an event page about an anti-quarantine protest in Michigan. He said that kind of thing was "harmful misinformation" and Facebook "will take that down."[18] According to company spokesman Andy Stone, the purge was justified because "events that defy government's guidance on social distancing aren't allowed on Facebook."[19]

Does that mean Facebook intends to side with *all* government guidance? Will they start trashing event pages for protests against Trump executive orders? Of course not. Facebook, along with most other Big Tech platforms, will continue to do all they can to support progressives. Nobody expects otherwise.

In early May, Knut M. Wittkowski, who specialized in biostatistics and epidemiology for twenty years at Rockefeller University, posted a video on YouTube. He offered sane and sober arguments against the American lockdown. YouTube memory-holed it.[20] In April, when Wittkowski first began speaking out, his former employer felt compelled to respond, announcing that his views "do not represent the views of The Rockefeller University, its leadership, or its faculty."[21]

Now, that normally goes without saying. We're not aware of any university that says their faculty speak for it. But in the age of social mania, many universities fear the diverse and critical dialog that used to be the essence of higher education. Evidently, Rockefeller University is one of them.

Many powerful institutions push "diversity"—except when it comes to diversity of viewpoint. It isn't only conservatives who see this. More and more academics from across the political spectrum are recognizing the damage this groupthink does to universities. Heterodox Academy was formed in 2015 to address the problem. By the thousands, its members have all declared, "I am concerned that many academic fields and universities currently lack sufficient viewpoint diversity."[22]

Big Tech has the same problem. But the fact that Big Tech leans left politically doesn't explain why they went into overdrive with the coronavirus. The press may have an incentive to hype fear, but so far as we know, hyping fears of viral infection isn't a key plank of progressive thought. Why, then?

Here's our theory: it's the same weird dynamic with expertise we've already seen. Big Tech is crowded with experts. The days of Bill Gates, Steve Jobs, and Susan Wojcicki working out of garages are mostly over (Wojcicki's garage was the first office of Google's Larry Page and Sergey Brin). These days, most high-level software engineers and tech business leaders come with academic credentials. Professors, researchers, and bureaucrats at places like WHO are themselves credentialed.

There's nothing wrong with credentials, of course. For the most part they do certify advanced knowledge in a field. Wojcicki absolutely knows the business and marketing of search engines and video streaming. If she's like most non-medical experts, though, she didn't know the difference between a coronavirus and a rhinovirus before 2020. Why would she? Outside medicine, no one cared, until recently.

Yet YouTube chose to become an arbiter on such questions. We doubt the company hired a team of virologists, pulmonologists, and epidemiologists to help them consider which videos to purge and which to keep and boost. So Wojcicki had to appeal to an outside source. But which one?

Why not *the best*? The best would be that group with the highest official credentials. At the global level, that's WHO. No, WHO isn't a brain trust of the smartest people in the world. It's a UN bureaucracy. But it's recognized the world over as *official*. Why not side with them on controversies related to the pandemic? If WHO turns out to be wrong on some of them, YouTube has a great excuse. If they turn out to be right, then YouTube will have made the right call.

It isn't mainly about being factually right or wrong. It's more about being visibly aligned with the right people. And more than *that*, it's about being seen to disapprove of the wrong people. It's called virtue signaling. The right people are those who occupy the highest positions in the intellectual establishment; the wrong people are those who criticize those right people.

It doesn't matter whether you think of journalists or tech leaders or Wikipedia editors as intellectuals. What matters is that they think of themselves that way. That's why they align themselves so slavishly with the consensus view of the intellectual establishment. On controversy after controversy, they prove that their imagined association with the big thinkers matters to them far more than getting it right.

With few exceptions, even the big thinkers think this way (hence the need for Heterodox Academy). The very elites who, if they had the courage, could balance the thinking of other elites instead end up in a mutually affirming dance. In this way, experts tend to reinforce a web of orthodox views across a multitude of fields.

But pull one thread and the whole thing unravels. This is why, when an outsider comes along and picks at a strand, the web-builders of the club of intellectual orthodoxy scream "Denier!" The braying is especially abusive if the outsider is uncredentialed. Spiders from the highest levels inhabit the center of the web, and the outsider is a real threat, like a giant bumbling grasshopper.

That's why YouTube couldn't just promote WHO. It had to purge videos that contradicted WHO's story of the day. It—and Facebook and the rest of the social media giants—had to promote only "respectable" content and purge the dissenters.

This is what happened to Drs. Erickson and Massihi, as we have seen. They had credentials, but by opposing orthodoxy they proved themselves to be the wrong kind of people. They had data and smarts, but they weren't club members. All the right people were (by definition) deferring to the highest health authorities.

Ditto for Aaron Ginn, a young Silicon Valley "growth hacker" interested in politics and tech policy. Drawing on stats from Johns Hopkins, he wrote a critique of the lockdown on Medium, the online magazine that claims to "encourage ideas that come from anywhere." It was surprisingly good, considering Ginn's lack of expertise. It soon got millions of views and inspired a healthy online debate.

Then an official infectious disease expert, Carl Bergstrom of the University of Washington, launched a nasty Twitter tirade against it. He said Ginn's piece was like "Shakespeare run through google translate into Japanese, then translated back to English by someone who'd never heard of Shakespeare." That's the kind of thing you say when you desperately want to oppose something but can't come up with a good argument. Anyone who had read the piece knew the charge was absurd. Ginn's piece was lucid and analytical. No matter. Medium pulled it down thirteen hours after it had gone up. Twitter dutifully added a warning to tweets about it. Other UW professors used it as an example of social media "misinformation" in a piece in the *Washington Post*.[23]

Medium then posted a piece by another Silicon Valley growth hacker, Tomás Pueyo. He argued that the coronavirus was far worse than most people thought. His article got boosts from Steven Pinker and the *New York Times*. BuzzFeed dubbed it the "defining piece on the outbreak of COVID-19."[24] Pueyo had no more expertise than Ginn, and it was factually wrong to boot, but he was on the right side. His piece is still up at Medium.

Again, it's your alignment that makes you right, not your credentials or the quality of your arguments. Take Knut Wittkowski, for example, one of the victims of YouTube censorship mentioned above. He's the former head of Biostatistics, Epidemiology and Research Design at Rockefeller University's Center for Clinical and Translational Science. He has a Ph.D. in computer science from the University of Stuttgart and a Doctor of Science degree in medical biometry from the University of Tübingen, both top German universities. He has as much expertise as anyone from WHO. But he was a staunch critic of the lockdowns and the logic behind them. That made him one of the wrong people.

UK-based Journey Pictures posted a hard-hitting video interview with him, giving him ample time to make his case for herd immunity over lockdowns. After it went viral, they posted a follow-up. Guess what happened to the first video? We don't need to tell you. You get it.

Experts who weren't censored (so far as we know) were blasted for bucking the party line. These included Stanford professor John Ioannidis, who published a study suggesting that the bug was more widespread than case testing revealed.[25] He and his team sampled people in Santa Clara County, California and discovered that the infection rate was indeed higher.

This should have been neither surprising nor controversial. Yet it was. True, Ioannidis and his team weren't offering the final word on the coronavirus, only an early and helpful look at the progress of the disease. But what happened, as the *New York Times* described it, was "the academic version of a roast."[26] Scientists and academics treated Ioannidis and his co-authors as if they had committed sacrilege. They went well beyond normal and helpful criticisms of the study's details, stooping to personal attacks in the cesspool of social media, which celebrated with its usual piling-on ceremony to discredit heretics.[27]

Media were incensed when critics of the shutdown quoted the study. Then came "revelations" from a "whistle-blower" that part of the study had been funded by a non-government entity. That damned the study beyond all hope. *The Nation* said that Stanford University—where Ioannidis is professor of medicine, health research, and biomedical data science—had "lost its soul."[28]

This is how the cult of expertise works. It's not about genuine smarts, careful science, or following the evidence where it leads. It's about the authority that comes from being a card-carrying member of the *official* club. Oppose the club, and you lose your card. There is an absurd idea that government money is pure and private money is tainted. And then there's the exception to this rule: any private individual with deep enough pockets to fund the club gets honorary membership. Bill Gates's foundation is the second largest donor to WHO after the United States,[29] so Gates is enlightened.

The social media giants propped up people who were on the side of a manufactured consensus, whether or not they were experts. And they suppressed people who were on the other side, whether or not they were experts. This made the pandemic panic not just scary, but creepy.

CHAPTER 5

RUSH TO LOCKDOWN

Democracy is the theory that the common people know
what they want, and deserve to get it good and hard.

—H. L. Mencken[1]

Politicians aren't immune to the symbiotic cult of expertise among media, social media platforms, and official experts. They're just as likely as tech CEOs to swoon before high-placed experts. Even those with partial immunity, like President Trump, can't ignore them when the press boosts their signals to the public. If polls show that voters are panicked, then presidents, governors, and mayors know that the public must see them doing something—*anything*—to fix the problem. By mid-March, most Americans wanted government action, good and hard.[2]

The belief that governments can and should fix every major problem is more pronounced on the political left than on the right. But given the circumstances, probably any occupant of the White House would have favored a lockdown, and most governors would have done the same. After all, most governments of most countries in the world responded in this way. That suggests that the cause of the pandemic panic transcended politics.

Indeed, the public panic was already well underway when politicians, sensing the groundswell, began competing for top prize in the "most serious response" category.

Some of them embraced their new powers with gusto. As we mentioned in our introduction, Philippine president Rodrigo Duterte ordered the police and military to kill citizens who defied the lockdown.[3]

Police in India were far more humane. In some places, they would drive around in their scooters and whack violators on the head.[4]

Here in the United States we settled for fines and imprisonment. Washington, D.C. mayor Muriel Bowser threatened residents with "90 days in jail and a $5,000 fine" if they left home during the crisis.[5] States issued similar threats to businesses. Vermont ordered Walmart and Target to stop selling non-essential items, such as clothing and electronics, in their stores.[6]

We won't belabor the point; you have your own stories. What we found perplexing was that, at first, few people opposed these restrictions. On the contrary: more often than not, the public took part, and even led the way.

SNITCHING

Rather than protesting government overreach, people around the world turned their neighbors in for bucking the lockdown. On March 30, Brendon O'Neill in Spiked warned of a second viral sickness spreading through Britain—"the sickness of snitching."[7]

As the title of one report put it, "Germans Snitch on Neighbours Flouting Virus Rules, in Echo of the Stasi Past." The reporter explained that "Munich police took up to 150 calls every day last week from citizens reporting alleged breaches of corona rules."[8]

Taiwan handled the crisis better than most countries. But there were still pockets of nuttiness in the country. For instance, the Taipei City Government offered rewards to those who reported mask litterers (Taiwanese wear a lot of masks).[9]

In the United States, Los Angeles mayor Eric Garcetti tried to undercut the social stigma attached to snitching. "You know the old expression about snitches," he said. "Well in this case they get rewards."[10] And it wasn't just neighbor ratting out neighbor. It was tribe snitching on tribe. One headline ran, "Coronavirus Delaware: Police Authorized to Pull Over Out-of-State Drivers during Pandemic."[11]

We didn't reach communist cutthroat levels of citizen spying. But there was a lot of snitching. One of us watched it daily on the neighborhood chat board, NextDoor. Neighbors ratted out neighbors for taking a second walk outdoors, for not social distancing, and for suspicions of other unsanctioned activities.

In a matter of weeks, the faint fear of death turned millions of us into cry-bullies.

WHY WE WENT ALONG

Why did the American public go along? It's one thing for us to decide it would be best to work from home and avoid large crowds. But it's quite another for cities and states to order us not to go to work or church, or even to leave our houses, and to arrest us if we don't comply. States can do this legally only in the most extreme emergencies. Most Americans had never witnessed anything like it—even in the middle of a hurricane. And yet, for the most part, we went along.

Millions of people were scared for themselves, but that was only part of the story. What made all the difference was this: we thought the lives of *other* people were at stake.

Your right to swing your fist, it's said, ends at your neighbor's nose. That's because your neighbor has the same rights you have, no more and no fewer. We so quickly surrendered our rights during the pandemic panic because the boundary between fist and nose got blurred. Most of us know the length of our arms and the distance to our neighbors' noses. But what if in exercising your right to visit the mall you inadvertently exhale infectious virus particles? Where's the cut-off? What if some of those particles find their way into the noses of others and infect them? What if those people go on to infect others unaware, and thousands of people die as a result? Your exercise of your liberties could be a death sentence for countless others.

"We're at war with a deadly virus," President Trump told Americans on March 31. "Success in this fight will require the full absolute measure of our collective strength, love, and devotion. It's very important. Each of us has the power through our own choices and actions to save American lives and rescue the most vulnerable among us."[12]

Powerful stuff. More than enough to suppress the liberty-loving hackles of most Americans, at least for a while. It's one thing to defend your right to religion and peaceable assembly. But what if your presence at church were to cause an infection that kills the eighty-five-year-old woman sitting in front of you?

As Senator Ted Cruz put it, "This crisis has shown us the character of the American people. We have seen that Americans of all walks of life are ready and willing to make sacrifices for the public good, to help stop the spread of this virus."[13]

The danger went beyond spreading the virus. The first justification for "social distancing" was to "flatten the curve"—to slow the spread of the infection in order to reduce pressure on the health care system. Maybe you weren't at much risk of death. But if you became sick enough to go to the hospital, you might need a bed, doctor, nurses, medicine, and equipment that could otherwise have saved the life of an elderly man.

Weirdly, by mid-March, avoiding others became our prime directive. "Proximity is usually associated with intimacy, and distance with strangeness," noted one anthropologist at the height of the frenzy. "The public challenge at the moment is that we must learn to express our care and concern by maintaining distance, which is counter-intuitive."[14]

This logic extended even to those who, at other times, would risk their lives to care for others. "It is one thing to make a martyr of one's self," noted Catholic priest and theologian Thomas Joseph White, "and another thing to eradicate a nursing home in the process. In a case like this, priests may only minister to those who are infected if they themselves are taking sufficient precautions not to infect others."[15] This was an acute problem for Catholics. Sermons and prayers can be delivered online. But sacraments can only be administered in person.

As a result, there's always some chance that a priest will infect someone. In the Catholic practice of communion, priests place consecrated hosts in hundreds, even thousands, of hands and mouths every week. They empty the chalice after communion by *drinking* what is left. The whole operation is a germophobe's nightmare. Most Catholics, and priests, take it in stride. They stay home or at least keep their distance if they're sick. They use hand sanitizer during flu season.

Suspending public Masses, confessions, and baptisms, then, only makes sense if the risk is extreme. For instance, if there's a highly contagious and uniquely deadly virus that would probably find its way into a chalice. Should Masses be cancelled if the case fatality rate of a virus is 1 percent? A tenth of a percent? A hundredth of a percent? It's hard, if not impossible, to say. But it's no surprise that church closures and stay-at-home orders, to name only two responses, were based on the early, apocalyptic, and wildly inaccurate, predictions about the coronavirus. That's how authorities persuaded even most priests that they had a duty to refrain from administering the sacraments—something they would not agree to even in a time of war, persecution, or mass starvation.

By mid-April, when doomsday didn't come, some started to question whether the risk justified the response. Opinion was sharply divided. On April 17, the *Washington Post* covered "right-wing" protests against the lockdowns in Michigan, Minnesota, and Virginia. "I call these people the modern-day Rosa Parks," reported the *Post*, quoting conservative economist Steve Moore. "They are protesting against injustice and a loss of liberties."[16] That earned Moore his Two Minutes Hate on Twitter. *New York Magazine* columnist Mark Harris summed up the sentiment: "I'll never forget the day Rosa Parks got on the bus with a submachine gun and refused to wear a mask because of freedom."[17] Others claimed the protesters had forfeited their right to health care, and even wished sickness and death upon them.

But peaceful protests are as American as apple pie. Imagine any other scenario. What if the president, governors, and mayors made us all close our businesses and churches and stay home because we take too many risks when we drive, work, or play in the park? We never would have tolerated it. There would have been huge bipartisan protests from the Atlantic to the Pacific. Conservatives would have bristled at the loss of liberty, and liberals would have denounced the fascists in the White House and the state houses.

As it was, however, most of us complied and self-enforced—for months.

Why? Because we believed the restrictions weren't just for our good. They were for the sake of others. The pandemic panic took hold because it appealed not just to our vices—our fear and petty partisanship—but to our virtues—to our love of elderly parents and grandparents and fellow Americans. As in jiu jitsu, authorities used our moral weight to hoist us by our own petards.

We'll show later why this move wasn't fair play. If we all had grasped how much harm the panicked lockdowns would do to others, we surely would have been less compliant.

PANDEMIC PANIC

If you were trapped in a simulation, as in *The Matrix*, could you tell? Would you notice the random glitch in your field of vision, the pixelated patch of sky, the repeating loop of video when you were jogging in your neighborhood? Or would you miss it, or explain it away, or just play along?

Change the scenario. Imagine that you were subject to a global campaign of psychological warfare. Every source of information seemed to confirm the same frightening story, and to appeal to the instinct for fear buried deep in your soul. But it was all misleading you. How would you tell? What strategy would you use to snap yourself out of it, to resist, to seek the truth, however unpleasant?

Would you miss it, or explain it away, or just play along?

Early in the last century, a million Europeans died from tuberculosis every year. In a few short months in 1918, as many as fifty million died from the Spanish flu. The two world wars led to over a hundred million deaths. None of these events shut down the global economy or led to compulsory stay-at-home orders around the world. None of them led the free world to empty churches and synagogues. And yet, in 2020, we did all those things—subjecting ourselves to the biggest social experiment the world has ever seen.

There were good reasons for skepticism, even at the beginning. And there is now overwhelming evidence that we fell under the spell—not of a conspiracy, but of a global social contagion. If you keep reading, you will no longer be able to miss it. Then you'll have a choice to make: face it, explain it away, or keep playing along.

CHAPTER 6

UNTANGLING THE NUMBERS

If you torture data long enough, it will confess to anything.

—*Ronald Coase*[1]

Assigning causes of death is a messy business. Hospital doctors with elderly patients beset by "comorbidities" face the dilemma every day. You have a ninety-year-old patient who dies. He had type 2 diabetes, angina, high blood pressure, and severe arthritis, and came to the emergency room the night before with flu symptoms. What do you put on the death certificate? There will typically be an immediate cause of death along with intermediate causes, underlying causes, and many complicating factors. Do you refer the patient for an autopsy, which is costly and time-consuming? Or do you forgo that, since the death was natural and imminent?

With the new coronavirus, politics made such choices even messier. The experts who had sounded the planet-wide alarm about the coronavirus and advised draconian shutdowns to fight it surely knew that they'd be blamed if it turned out to be a false alarm. So they had good reason, conscious or not, to exaggerate COVID-19 deaths. And if the real numbers ended up far below the forecasts, they would want to credit the shutdowns for the drop. The last thing they'd want to do is admit a colossal "oops."

WHO declared the COVID-19 outbreak a "Public Health Emergency of International Concern" on January 30.[2] On March 11, they upgraded that to a pandemic.[3] Two weeks later, on March 25, they issued guidelines for designating cases as COVID-19. By these new rules, a patient with a fever and a cough who required hospitalization would be classified among "suspected cases of COVID-19" if the attending clinician thought that best fit the symptoms.[4] Furthermore, "a *probable* case is a *suspected* case for whom the report from laboratory testing for the COVID-19 virus is inconclusive."[5] You read that right. The protocol called for suspected cases to be elevated to probable cases if the test result was *inconclusive*.

Disease-control groups throughout the world pressed these rules onto doctors. On April 8, a local public school district alerted one of us that a teacher had been diagnosed with COVID-19. "The teacher…visited an emergency room on Sunday, April 5, 2020, where he was diagnosed by a doctor. The teacher was not tested; however, he was diagnosed by the doctor based upon his symptoms." This was a bizarre standard—particularly when you consider that at that time 80 percent of tests on people with symptoms were coming back negative.[6]

The standards for cause of death were equally lax. In the United States, the CDC changed the rules mid-stream, declaring in early April that doctors could list COVID-19 as the official cause of death without a test.[7] The change led to a spike in official deaths from the coronavirus.[8] Stories started appearing of families questioning how COVID-19 had appeared on the death certificates of loved ones, without evidence.[9]

Classification of deaths was a moving target throughout the pandemic. Naturally, the press fixed on any excuse to paint a grimmer picture. For example, COVID Tracking at *The Atlantic* reported 91,287 coronavirus deaths in the United States on May 22, almost 24 percent higher than the 73,639 figure the CDC was reporting at the same time. This discrepancy became consistent by early May, as Figure 6.1 shows. The press often defended the elevated figures on the grounds of delayed official recording by the CDC. According to the CDC, their numbers "provide the most complete and accurate picture of lives lost to COVID-19."[10]

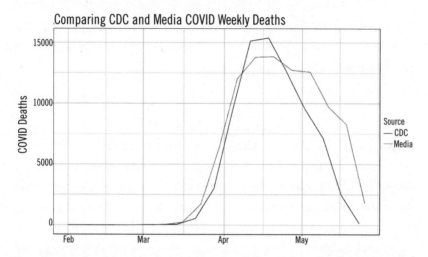

Figure 6.1. Comparison of weekly COVID-19 death counts from the CDC (Death Counts for Coronavirus Disease: https://www.cdc.gov/nchs/nvss/vsrr/covid19/index. htm) and the COVID Tracking Project (associated with *The Atlantic*; https:// covidtracking.com), through May 26, 2020.

In the UK, pathology professor John Lee explained that his country had not previously recorded the pathogens leading to death by respiratory failure (a common cause of death) on death certificates "unless the illness is a rare 'notifiable disease.'"[11] Until recently, the list of those special diseases excluded common seasonal viruses, such as the flu and previous coronaviruses. Instead, it included the really scary pathogens—anthrax, the plague, and so forth.

Adding COVID-19 to this list was a self-fulfilling prophecy: it inflated the count of COVID-19 deaths. As Dr. Lee put it, "Making COVID-19 notifiable might give the appearance of it causing increasing numbers of deaths, whether this is true or not." By the new rules, whatever the true cause of death, once a patient tests positive, hospital staff "*have* to record the COVID-19 designation on the death certificate—contrary to usual practice for most infections of this kind." This conflates dying *with* the virus and dying *from* the virus.

In the United States, the CDC issued guidelines that were just as confusing. No wonder Dr. Deborah Birx is reported to have said at a Coronavirus Task Force meeting in May, "There is nothing from the CDC that I can trust."[12] The press, of course, welcomed inflated numbers and even added their own inflation.

How Deadly Is It?

So, let's set aside the headlines, which are blind guides, and see if we can answer the simple question: How dangerous is the new coronavirus to public health? Is it often the *sole* cause of a death, like Ebola, which kills about half the people it infects, including the healthy?[13] Or does it mainly contribute to death among unhealthy people, like the seasonal flu virus?

A real nightmare virus would be as deadly as Ebola and as contagious as the flu. Such a bug would infect around 20 percent of the population and kill half the people it infects—about *eight hundred million* deaths worldwide, over 30 million of those in the U.S. Something like this happened when Europe lost about a third of its population to a bacterial pandemic (the bubonic plague) from 1347 to 1352.

In fact, the coronavirus is neither like the bubonic plague nor Ebola, which both kill large swathes of people, healthy and unhealthy alike. Like the seasonal flu, it mostly contributes to the deaths of people who are old or already ill from other causes. When the coronavirus kills, it does so by causing severe pneumonia, which ultimately leads to respiratory failure. Most people who catch the flu or the coronavirus recover, though. Both viruses can work their way from the upper to the lower respiratory tract to trigger pneumonia. But a strong immune response usually clears the infection before this happens.

This is how typical flu viruses differ from the much more lethal variants such as as the Spanish flu. A normal flu season claims mostly elderly people because of their weaker immune systems and other health problems.[14] But the elderly can actually have an advantage when it comes to much rarer but more deadly flu variants that appear only a few times per century. Why? Because they've lived through more of these rare epidemics. Their immune systems may be more sluggish, but they tend to carry antibodies from prior infections. That's why rare versions of the flu kill a disproportionate number of healthy young people. The 1918 Spanish flu, for example, hit people aged eighteen to thirty-five years old.[15] The 2009 swine flu seemed to target the twenty-five-to-forty-nine age group.[16]

A good way to assess a new cause of pneumonia, then, is to compare it to previous causes. Are the victims much younger and healthier than usual victims of pneumonia? That would be a warning flag. If, on the other hand, the pneumonia deaths fit the usual demographic profile, then there's less cause for concern.

The average age of people who die of pneumonia in the U.S. is about seventy-six years.[17] Over 80 percent of them already had serious health problems.[18] One study found that nearly half of pneumonia victims had coronary artery disease.[19] More than a third had kidney or liver disease, and over a quarter had cancer.

How does the new coronavirus compare? A March 23 report in the *Journal of the American Medical Association* offered the first clue.[20] It was a detailed review of the medical records for 355 COVID-19 victims in Italy. Victims averaged 79.5 years of age and were in poor health. More than a third had diabetes, and just under a third had ischemic heart disease. A quarter had atrial fibrillation. A fifth had active cancer, and over a sixth had either dementia or a history of stroke. Of the 355 people, only *three* were in good health before catching the coronavirus.

Data from the United States paint a similar picture. As of May 20, the age at death by coronavirus averaged 76.2 years.[21] As in Italy, these were predominantly unhealthy people. In New York, where deaths were highest in the United States, 89.1 percent of the victims had suffered from at least one serious health problem before contracting the virus.[22] There were exceptions, of course, but as a rule, coronavirus victims look very much like the usual victims of pneumonia: elderly and sickly. That's why the coronavirus hit nursing homes so hard.[23]

The CDC reported an average of 2.5 *non*-COVID conditions listed on the certificates for deaths attributed to the coronavirus.[24] In fact, COVID-19 was the sole cause listed for *only 7 percent* of these deaths. More perplexingly, "intentional and unintentional injury, poisoning and other adverse events" were listed as a causes for several thousand deaths attributed to COVID-19. That's a small fraction of the total, but it shows a systematic problem with how data were handled during the pandemic. The CDC does strive for accuracy in the long run, but it takes time to deliver that. When the press is clamoring for bad-news headlines on an hourly basis, they're bound to get frustrated with the lengthy process of finalizing the data on deaths. So, they cut corners and put out half-baked numbers in a hurry.

Figure 6.2 shows how the highly imperfect counts of coronavirus deaths in 2020[25] compare to pneumonia deaths in 2018 and total deaths in 2018 in several states.[26] In only three of them—New York, New Jersey,

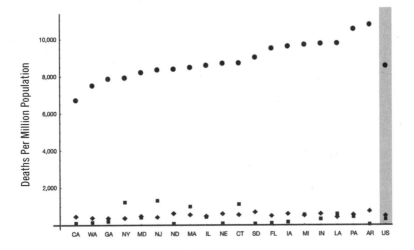

Figure 6.2. Comparison of COVID-19-attributed deaths in various states in 2020 (squares) to 2018 figures for total deaths (circles) and pneumonia deaths (diamonds). COVID-19 death counts are accurate as of May 31, 2020. Data source: https:// covidtracking.com/data.

and Connecticut—were the coronavirus deaths a lot higher than the pneumonia deaths. Elsewhere, the deaths attributed to the virus were near or even below the number attributed to pneumonia in 2018. In no state did the virus cause more than a sliver of the normal annual deaths.

Nevertheless, in some states COVID-19 took more lives in 2020 than pneumonia did in 2018 (a relatively bad pneumonia year). These really are excess deaths. Despite all the messiness of the counting, then, the coronavirus clearly killed many people before they otherwise would have died.

CASES, INFECTIONS, DEATHS, CONFUSION

Although it wasn't helpful for the public to become obsessed with death rates, they are a standard aspect of epidemiology. Estimated fatality rates can be based either on infections or cases. The first (the infected-fatality rate, or IFR) is simple in principle: take the total number of people who have died *from* the bug and divide it by the total number infected by it. That's easier said than done, because there's no easy way to count the infections. Test results tell us a certain number, but that number always depends on another, highly variable number: how many people have been tested.

The case-fatality rate (CFR), in contrast, is simple in practice but more ambiguous in definition. The number of dead is the same, but now that's divided by the number of infected people who have become "cases." What is a case? Well, someone who shows up at the hospital to be treated, usually. But cases in the COVID-19 pandemic weren't quite like that. They were a mix of people who showed up at hospitals and those who showed up at testing sites. Some didn't show up at all. That is, some sick people were probably too afraid to seek treatment, so they stayed home and were never counted. How many? Nobody knows.

Early estimates of the case-fatality rate of the new coronavirus were 0.3 to 1.3 percent. Better estimates of the infection-fatality rate put it at 0.15 to 0.26 percent (see below, page 65).

Figure 6.3 shows how badly the reported case counts underestimate the real number of people infected by the virus. The dark line at the

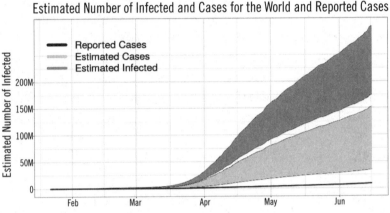

Figure 6.3. Total reported COVID-19 cases globally by date, compared to the estimated total number of cases and infections. The estimates are derived using actual infection and case rates given by the CDC and other sources. This shows that the reported cases do not come close to measuring the true extent of the spread of the coronavirus.

bottom shows total reported cases worldwide, which we know must be too low if the estimated case-fatality rates are anywhere near the mark. The lighter grey envelope estimates the total number of actual cases (given the 0.3 percent to 1.3 percent range for case-fatality rates). There are far more actual cases than reported cases—anywhere from 5 to 21 times as many. The total number of actual cases by May 27 was anywhere from 25 to 120 million people. That is, about 0.3 percent to 1.6 percent of the world's population had experienced symptoms or were otherwise cases by that date.

The dark grey envelope shows the estimated total number of infected people worldwide, by date, using the estimated infection-fatality rates of 0.15 percent to 0.26 percent. The 0.15 percent (highest line) IFR gives the largest estimate of total infections. This makes sense, since for a given number of deaths, more infections drive infection-fatality rates lower. The estimated number of infected people is 25 to 43 times higher than the reported cases. This will matter when we consider what the media did with reported cases. We estimate the number of actual infections by May 27 to have been between 140 and 240 million people. That is, about 1.8 percent to 3 percent of the world's population had been infected by that date.

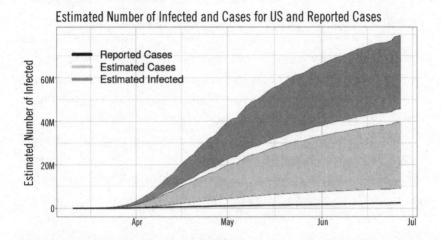

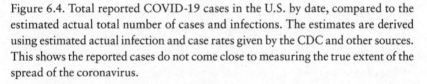

Figure 6.4. Total reported COVID-19 cases in the U.S. by date, compared to the estimated actual total number of cases and infections. The estimates are derived using estimated actual infection and case rates given by the CDC and other sources. This shows the reported cases do not come close to measuring the true extent of the spread of the coronavirus.

Figure 6.4 makes the same comparison for the United States. As before, the bottom dark line shows the total reported cases. The lighter gray envelope represents estimates of total cases assuming 0.3 to 1.3 percent CFRs. Again, we estimate the actual total cases to be about 5 to 19 times higher than the reported cases. The total number of actual cases by May 27 was anywhere from 8 to 30 million Americans. That is, about 2.4 percent to 9.1 percent of the U.S. population had experienced symptoms or were otherwise cases by that date.

The darker gray envelope represents estimates of total infected people, assuming 0.15 to 0.26 percent IFRs. So, the number of infected would have been about *twenty-two to thirty-eight times higher* than the reported case numbers. The number of actual infections would have been anywhere from 37 to 62 million people. That is, about 11 percent to 19 percent of the U.S. population had been infected by May 27.

Recall that all these estimates rely on the truth of reported death totals. If those are too high, then the estimated cases and infections will also be too high. Still, they help us estimate the number of true cases and infections, which is good to know in itself. They also help frame what the press and authorities did with cases and testing. As deaths went up in March and April, they reported on these day by day, hour by hour. The message was clear: unless you submit to the constraints, it's only a matter of time before the bug kills you or someone you love.

Then, by late April, the daily deaths started dropping. But this good news got less coverage than the previous bad news; instead, the press now spent more time reporting *cases*. In mid-May, NPR noted a "spike" in cases in Texas meatpacking plants after the state began restoring liberties.[27] *The Hill* seemed delighted to report on "rising cases" in Texas, North Carolina, and Arizona after those states loosened the reins.[28] Every new state that opened up became a new media target.

Of course, the easiest way to end new reported cases would be to stop testing for them. The opposite is also true: to get more reported cases, do more tests. Figures 6.3 and 6.4 expose the trick nicely. Back in March, the number of infected people, or cases, was much higher than reported figures. More testing would have revealed them. And lo and behold, when more tests were available and more people were tested, more infections were reported! It wasn't simply that more people were getting infected—it was that more infections were being detected.[29]

If there's a spike in new cases when the deaths are plummeting, it's almost certainly because there's more testing. And make no mistake: deaths were plummeting through May. Figure 6.5 shows the CDC's provisional COVID-19 death counts in the U.S. by week for various age groups. Across all ages, deaths were dropping before the end of April. One good explanation for the decline is the onset of herd immunity. That happens when enough of the susceptible population has been infected to slow further deadly infections. Lockdowns were meant to spread out ("flatten") the infection curves. This would also spread out the death curves. We'll take a critical look at whether they worked in chapter 9. In any case, the virus had largely run its deadly course by the end of June.

Forest fires often follow a similar trajectory. They spread fast when a dry-wooded region is mostly unburned, but at some point they run out of trees. At that point, an honest press would report that the fire is contained and largely out. Of course, reporters could find little pockets of fire and set up their cameras there for a while. That's what the media did with COVID-19. Well into July, they tried to keep the COVID flames burning by chasing case numbers.

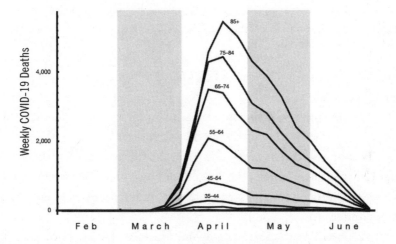

Figure 6.5. Weekly deaths attributed to COVID-19 in the U.S., as reported by the CDC through the week ending June 27, 2020. Labels show age ranges for the upper six curves. The curve for deaths at 25–34 years of age is visible below the one for 35–44. Deaths among people under 25 are plotted in a single curve, with numbers too small to be seen here.

On May 20, according to Worldometer, the globally reported COVID-19 deaths were 329,732, and the reported cases were 5,090,064. What we're calling the case-fatality rate, then, was 6.5 percent. The reported deaths in the United States, according to the Covid Tracking Project, were 87,472, and reported cases were 1,542,309. Using those

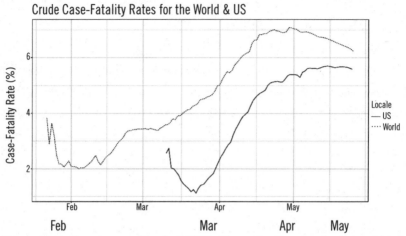

Figure 6.6. Daily estimates of crude COVID-19 case-fatality rates for the world and the United States, through May 21.

numbers, the case-fatality rate was 5.7 percent. Which is right, 6.5 percent or 5.7 percent?

Neither. Figure 6.6 shows how estimates of these case fatality rates varied from day to day for the world and for the U.S. as the pandemic ran its course. If there's really one true rate, then most of the daily estimates are wrong. In fact, they could *all* be wrong. This is why we've stressed that they are based on reported cases and deaths, and not actual cases and deaths.

If reported deaths are too high—for example, if many who died *with* and not *from* the virus were classified as COVID deaths—then the case-fatality rate will also be too high. Undercounting or under-reporting the actual cases would also make the rate too high. Both errors were probably occurring.

More relevant than the case-fatality rate is the infection-fatality rate. This is the number that might tell you how likely death is if you catch the virus—sort of. The two are quite different, though the press didn't always make the distinction. The coronavirus wasn't killing 5 to 7 percent of the people it infected in early May, as a naive reading of these figures might suggest. The limited testing wasn't revealing all infections. Most infected people weren't tested because they had few or no symptoms.

What's the real infection-fatality rate, then? At the time of writing, no one knows for sure. Experts using intelligent sampling of the data, such as verified autopsy reports, will estimate it later. Some studies have already commenced. One put the "infection-fatality" rate "of symptomatic patients" at a whopping 1.3 percent![30] But that's not a real infection-fatality rate; that's just another way to state the case-fatality rate. Why? Those who were infected but didn't have symptoms weren't counted in the study. Other studies yielded case-fatality estimates as low as 0.3 percent, which means the infection-fatality rates must have been lower still.[31] The case-fatality rate for the flu is about 0.1 percent. Based on those figures, we could say COVID-19 is three times deadlier than the flu—if you become a "case," that is. Right now, though, there's a lot of ambiguity about what makes a COVID-19 case.

What's certain is that the infection-fatality rate must be lower than the case-fatality rate. A study of asymptomatic rhinovirus infections, the most common cause of the common cold, estimated that "asymptomatic infection was four times as common as symptomatic infection." For MERS-CoV (a virus sort of like COVID-19, but much more common in children), on the other hand, asymptomatic cases were only 1 to 42 percent of symptomatic cases.[32] So if the COVID-19 case-fatality rate was around 0.3 percent to 1.3 percent, then, using the rhinovirus estimates as the lower bound and the larger MERS estimate for the upper bound, the infection-fatality rate was likely around 0.15 percent to 0.26 percent.

The infection-fatality rate for the ordinary flu depends on the particular strain, but common numbers used are 0.04 percent to 0.1 percent.[33] We could compare the 2009 swine flu pandemic, but it's a strained comparison, because the infection rate by age was nearly inverted from COVID-19. Swine flu went after the young, COVID-19 after the old. Swine flu spread easily. One study found the infection rate—the total number of people who caught the bug—was 39 percent of three to nineteen year olds, but only 0.77 percent for sixty-plus-year-olds.[34] That same study found an overall (age-averaged) infection-fatality rate of 0.007 percent. The CDC produced similar estimates.[35]

We can derive precise fatality numbers from the natural lockdown experiment of the *Princess* cruise ship, where all 3,770 passengers and crew were quarantined. (Note, though, that this might not match how the disease would act in a normal population.) According to the Japanese Self Defense Force, "The average age of the patients was 68 years, and the number of men and women was almost half. Crew passengers are mainly in their 30s to 50s. Passengers were mainly in their 70s."[36] There were 712 reported infections, for an infection rate of 19 percent. There were 13 deaths, for an infection-fatality rate of 1.8 percent—quite high, even when age is taken into account. But this was also the case-fatality rate, since all infections on the ship were treated as cases. The overall fatality rate (deaths per population) was 0.3 percent. But all of these figures must represent an upper bound, because of the close quarantine. It's not surprising that all the numbers are smaller in areas outside quarantines.

It also reminds us that neither the case-fatality rate nor the infection-fatality rate tells us much. The overall fatality rate better reveals the true danger of a virus. After all, not everybody catches the bug, not everybody who catches it gets sick, and not everybody who gets sick dies. But even the overall rate is crude, in that it doesn't distinguish the segments of a population by age or by prior health. So a number that applies to a population as a whole doesn't necessarily match *your* risk.

Past Pandemics

How, then, should we compare the lethality of the present pandemic with that of past ones? One decent measure would be the percentage of the world population killed.

This number also measures disruption: the higher the number killed, the greater impact on those left alive, and those yet to be born. The details of past pandemics are often uncertain, however.[37] The closer the events are to the present, the more we know. But even in the twentieth century, we may have rather crude estimates. Estimated deaths from the Spanish flu, for example, range from seventeen to almost sixty million.[38] Still, it makes sense to compare these events, especially the ones in the last few centuries, to the current pandemic.

In Table 6.5 we've put together the information for eighteen historically significant plagues, epidemics, and pandemics. The numbers for these in modern times are pretty accurate. The further back we go in time, the less certain they are. We only show events where the total number of deaths was reported to be at least a hundred thousand.[39]

Event	Date	World Deaths	Percent
Plague of Athens	429–426 BC	75–100 thousand	0.8
Antonine Plague	165–180 AD	5–10 million	3
Plague of Cyprian	258 AD	1 million	0.4
Plague of Justinian	541–542 AD	25–100 million	21
Japanese smallpox	735–737 AD	2 million	0.6
Black Death	1331–1353	75–100 million	21
Mexico smallpox epidemic	1520	5–8 million	1.4
Cocoliztli epidemic	1545–1548	5–15 million	0.2
Cocoliztli epidemic	1576–1580	2–2.5 million	0.4
Italian plague	1629–1631	280 thousand	0.05
Great Plague of London	1665–1666	100 thousand	0.02
Great Plague of Marseille	1720–1722	100 thousand	0.007
Persian Plague	1772	2 million	0.2
First cholera pandemic	1816–1826	100 thousand	0.009
Second cholera pandemic	1829–1851	100 thousand	0.008
Third cholera pandemic	1852–1860	1 million	0.008
Flu pandemic	1889–1890	1 million	0.06

Table 6.1. The percent killed worldwide for various diseases with death tolls of at least 100,000, up to the beginning of the twentieth century. World population figures for the percent calculation are from Wikipedia.[40]

History records many plagues without giving death counts. Only just over half of the noted epidemics have death tolls in the historical record.

Pandemics also happened less often in ancient days, since most people never wandered far from home. But concentrated populations still allowed for huge death tolls. The Antonine plague of 165–180 AD killed about 3 percent of the world population. An equivalent proportion today would be 231 million deaths (3 percent of 7.7 billion). About four centuries later came the Plague of Justinian, which took out approximately 21 percent of the world's population in about one year—the equivalent of 1.6 *billion* deaths in today's world! An event of that scale today would be ample cause for panic.

The only other recorded event of that magnitude is Europe's Black Death. Spread out over twenty years or so, it wiped out between seventy-five and one hundred million people. This again was about 21 percent of the world's population—an epic disaster.

There's a clear trend across time, with most of the events killing 1 percent or more of the world population happening in the Middle Ages or before. This could be due to recording bias. Whatever the reason, in modern times the only event to break 1 percent was the Mexico smallpox epidemic of 1520, which killed from 5 to 8 million. At that time there were about 480 million people on the planet. A similar event today would wipe out about 108 million.

Historical records don't list the flu as a major killer until 1889–1890, when it killed about a million people, or roughly 0.06 percent of the 1.6 billion people alive at that time. A comparable event today would claim 4.6 million lives.

Epidemics and pandemics since 1900 are listed in Table 6.6. The devastating smallpox plague lasted from 1877 to about 1977, a full century. It is thought to have claimed about five hundred million lives, an average of 0.3 percent killed per year for a hundred years.

Some scientists claim the HIV/AIDS outbreak began as early as 1920, though most of the deaths did not occur until the late 1970s and early 1980s. On average, in the previous century, HIV/AIDS killed about

Percent Worldwide	Deaths	Date	Event
0.007*	> 12 million	1855–1960	Bubonic plague pandemic
0.0002*	> 800 thousand	1899–1923	Sixth cholera pandemic
0.008*	1.5 million	1915–1926	Encephalitis lethargica pandemic
3	17–100 million	1918–1920	Spanish flu
0.07	2 million	1957–1958	Asian flu
0.3*	500 million	1877–1977	Smallpox
0.03	1 million	1968–1969	Hong Kong flu
0.02*	> 32 million	1920–Present	HIV/AIDS pandemic
0.009	152–575 thousand	2009–2010	Swine flu
0.004	400 thousand	2019–June, 2020	COVID-19

Table 6.2. Epidemics and pandemics with at least 100,000 dead since the beginning of the twentieth century. The percentages with asterisks are rough averages per year, as these represent events that occurred over multi-year spans. For example, smallpox killed an average of about 0.3 percent of all people per year from 1877 to 1977.

0.02 percent per year. The bubonic plague, caused by the same bacteria as the earlier Black Death, also ranged over a century: it began in 1855 and lasted until 1960, killing about twelve million people, mostly in India and China.

The other events were more localized in time. The Spanish flu is the most infamous, having killed anywhere from 17 to 58 million, with some estimates as high as 100 million. If the 58 million number is right, then that influenza outbreak killed 3 percent of the roughly 2 billion people alive. This would be 231 million in today's numbers!

Among the more recent influenza outbreaks, the Asian flu (1957–1958) killed about two million people, or 0.07 percent of the world population. There was no worldwide panic. The Hong Kong flu, in the 1968–1969 season, killed about 1 million people, or 0.03 percent of the population. Again, no worldwide panic.

SARS was a media event in 2002–2004, especially in Asia. There was widespread worry at the time, expressed by both official and unofficial sources, that this disease might cause major devastation. And yet it killed only 772 people—not enough to be included in our chart. Remember the mosquito-borne zika virus? It generated a flurry of headlines in 2015–2016, focused on dangers to pregnant women. It killed 53 people.

BETTER THE DEVIL YOU KNOW

WHO estimates that "up to 650 thousand people across the globe each year die from respiratory illnesses linked to flu," or .0083 percent of the world's population in a bad flu year.[41] Yet no one panics when it comes to this persistent killer, even in the worst years.

Since actual counting is impractical, the CDC instead estimates the number of symptomatic flu illnesses, hospitalizations, and deaths each year.[42] These estimates come from a model, so they're uncertain. The CDC puts bounds around a central estimate, within which they're 95 percent sure the correct number lies. This number is useful for gauging the quantity of needed medical services.

Figure 6.7 shows the estimated number of symptomatic flu infections for each flu season from 2011 to 2019.[43] As of April 4, 2020, the CDC closed out its preliminary estimates for the 2019–2020 flu season. Their estimate was thirty-one to forty-five million symptomatic illnesses,

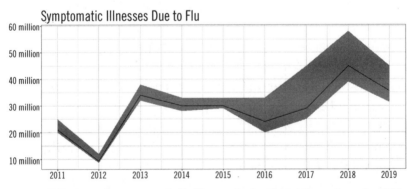

Figure 6.7. Estimated symptomatic flu illnesses in the United States from the 2011–2012 season to the 2019–2020 season. Estimates are plotted at the year when the season started (so the estimate for the 2019–2020 season is placed at 2019).

making this an average year.[44] The 2017–2018 season, in contrast, was a bad year for the flu. The estimate for that year was forty-five million symptomatic illnesses, with anywhere from thirty-nine to fifty-eight million possible. This means that 12 to 18 percent of the country suffered from the flu.

Next, in Figure 6.8, are flu hospitalizations over the same time period. By the end of May 2020, there had been an estimated 410,000–740,000 hospitalizations for the 2019–2020 season. Again, the 2017–2018 year was particularly bad. There were an estimated 810,000 hospitalizations, with the confidence range running from 620,000 to 1.4 million.

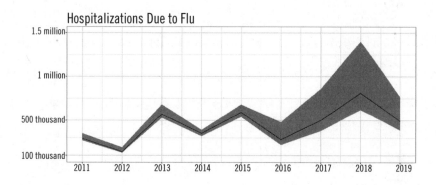

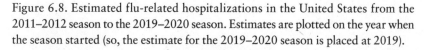

Figure 6.8. Estimated flu-related hospitalizations in the United States from the 2011–2012 season to the 2019–2020 season. Estimates are plotted on the year when the season started (so, the estimate for the 2019–2020 season is placed at 2019).

The flu puts lots of people in the hospital, including previously healthy people. In 2016, one of us (Jay Richards) ended up in the hospital with acute pneumonia and pleural effusion. My chest cavity filled up with sticky fluid, which caused my left lung, in effect, to stick to my ribs. I could barely breathe. As my wife drove me to the emergency room, I heard a choir sing (with no radio on) and was probably just a few hours from death. I spent days in intensive care, enduring procedures that didn't fix the problem. I finally had major surgery, which required the doctors to collapse my lung. I spent another week in the hospital afterwards, with three large tubes inside my chest cavity, and exiting my left side. The doctor only removed them on the day she discharged me. It took weeks to get off a cocktail of opioids, and months to fully recover. All of this started with a run-of-the-mill cold or flu. I was healthy and in my forties. Just think what the flu can do to old people in poor health!

Figure 6.9 shows the number of deaths attributed to the flu each year in the U.S. The median is about thirty-eight thousand. The estimate for the 2019–2020 season is twenty-four to sixty-two thousand deaths. Once again, the 2017–2018 year was especially bad. The best guess was sixty-one thousand killed (anywhere from forty-six to ninety-five thousand).

The 2019–2020 flu season was average-to-low in terms of deaths, as you can see in Figure 6.10. Flu deaths tend to start around the first of October. They quickly grow, peaking right around, or just after, the new year in bad seasons like 2014–2015 and 2017–2018, or around the beginning of March in average years. By mid-May, the flu is no longer a concern.

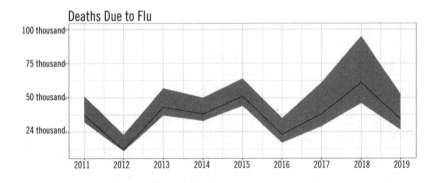

Figure 6.9. Estimated flu-related deaths in the U.S. from the 2011–2012 season to the 2019–2020 season. Estimates are plotted at the year when the season started (thus the estimate for the 2019–2020 season is placed at 2019). Data source: "Pneumonia and Influenza Mortality Surveillance from the National Center for Health Statistics Morality Surveillance System," CDC, https://gis.cdc.gov/grasp/fluview/mortality.html; "NCHSData 14 (5)," CDC, https://www.cdc.gov/flu/weekly/weeklyarchives2019-2020/data/NCHSData15.csv.

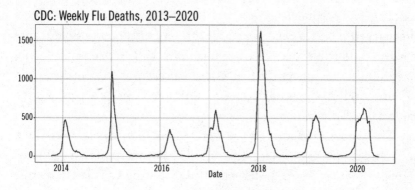

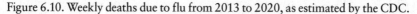

Figure 6.10. Weekly deaths due to flu from 2013 to 2020, as estimated by the CDC.

COVID-19 IN CONTEXT

COVID-19 will go down in history, but not for the number of deaths it caused, as you can see from Table 6.6 above. All death brings pain, but as far as historic pandemics go, the coronavirus was unremarkable. What was remarkable is how we reacted. The 2009 swine flu pandemic, which killed between 152,000 and 575,000 (as much as 0.009 percent of the world population), caused no panic. By the end of May 2020, COVID-19 might have claimed about as many as the swine flu.

The press covered the swine flu, but there was no worldwide panic. Perhaps it was social media that made the difference. Or perhaps it was the media's very different attitudes toward the occupants in the White House in 2009 and 2020.[45]

There has been a lot of confusion about causes of death among people infected with the coronavirus. Was the virus amplifying pre-existing health problems? That is, was it just one factor among others in hastening death in at-risk groups such as the elderly? If so, then we needed a way to count the extra deaths caused by the virus above those that would have occurred anyway. This was a problem with the data itself, quite apart from forecasts.

Yet even if COVID-19 really caused all the deaths associated with it, the virus won't rank among the deadliest disease agents. Indeed, we knew early on that most who catch it don't even show symptoms.

The new coronavirus won't rank high even among the deadliest preventable diseases. The World Health Organization estimates that malaria claimed the lives of approximately 1 million people, including 272,000 children under age five, in 2018 alone! But most of them died in Africa and Asia, cut off from prominent cable news shows and the Hollywood Twitterati.

The clamor to shut down the world in 2020 began before even ten thousand people worldwide—most of them advanced in years and suffering from other health problems—had died from COVID-19. Bernie Sanders, who often implied that Donald Trump was a fascist dictator, suddenly warmed to the idea of calling out the military in response to the virus.[46]

Whatever led to the unprecedented shutdown of the world economy and curtailment of rights in the coronavirus panic, it wasn't a historic number of deaths.

CHAPTER 7

BLIND MODELS

Quit trying to predict the future. You're having a hard enough time predicting the past.

—Edward C. Banfield's advice to social scientist James Q. Wilson[1]

Plenty of data about the new coronavirus was available early on, but as we've seen, it was a mess, especially when it came to teasing out causes, effects, and confounders. Governments ended up making calls based not on catastrophic numbers of present deaths, but on epidemiological models that predicted such numbers. These were educated guesses disguised as hard science. And, as it turned out, they weren't very good guesses.

HOW TO BET WRONG AND STILL WIN BIG

History shows that you will rarely lose your job making predictions if you're wrong in the right direction. On the other hand, you may well lose it if you're right in the wrong direction. Neither rulers nor subjects welcome the bearer of bad, but true, news. (Especially if it's bad news for power-grabbing elites.)

"I have been very jealous for the Lord, the God of hosts; for the people of Israel have forsaken thy covenant, thrown down thy altars, and slain thy prophets with the sword; and I, even I only, am left; and they seek my life, to take it away." (1 Kings 19:14, Revised Standard Version). So complained the Prophet Elijah to God, when he was fleeing for his life from Old Testament power-couple Ahab and Jezebel. Elijah predicted a drought: "Now Elijah the Tishbite, of Tishbe in Gilead, said to Ahab, 'As the Lord the God of Israel lives, before whom I stand, there shall be neither dew nor rain these years, except by my word.'" (1 Kings 17:1, Revised Standard Version). However right he was, no one wanted to hear what Elijah had to say. No one thanked him when the prophesied drought came to pass.

Being wrong in the right direction, though, often reaps reward. Early pandemic models indicated that only prompt and massive state action could save us. The models were wrong—way off—but they were wrong in the right direction. They gave politicians justification for taking over almost every aspect of citizens' lives. They gave the press clickbait galore. We're not assuming malice here. We assume that many of these folks were moved by concern and even love for others. The issue is one of incentives and human nature, not bad intentions.

Some models—naturally less exciting to reporters and less favored by experts pushing drastic mitigation efforts—said the coronavirus would be like most other viral outbreaks, probably like a really bad flu year. The virus would come and then it would go. Those scenarios suggested that the best strategy would be to protect the vulnerable while allowing the population at large to acquire herd immunity; extreme measures would likely do more harm than good.

But this was not what the leaders of most countries wanted to hear. Elites don't tend to welcome the news that the best thing they can do is stand aside, that their gifts are unwelcome and their interference may even cause harm. So they didn't hear it. The non-alarmist models were right in the wrong direction.

They favored instead the alarmist models, which were wrong in the right direction.

A Sorry Track Record

The historical record shows that those who are wrong in the right direction can be richly rewarded. Take Neil Ferguson, who headed the thirty-person COVID-19 Imperial College Response Team in the UK until he was caught violating his own advice during the lockdown. The *Financial Times* called Ferguson "a big name in epidemiological modelling." That's why his initial coronavirus model "sent a shockwave through the system in both the UK and the US, leading to the introduction of the present British policy of 'social distancing' and suppression, with its heavy economic and social costs for the public."[2]

Ferguson's is a career rich in the rewards of making wrong predictions in the right direction. In 2001, in response to the foot and mouth disease crisis in the UK, Ferguson's group created a model that called for a mass culling of animals. There were severe criticisms of his forecasts. It "has been claimed by experts such as Michael Thrusfield, professor of veterinary epidemiology at Edinburgh University, that Ferguson's modelling on foot and mouth was 'severely flawed' and made a 'serious error' by 'ignoring the species composition of farms,' and the fact that the disease spread faster between different species."[3] But Ferguson and his model prevailed. The cost of the decisions inspired by the model? Around ten billion pounds. Ferguson, so far as we can tell, suffered no loss as a result.

In the late 1990s, mad cow disease (bovine spongiform encephalopathy, BSE) was suspected of causing vCJD (variant Creutzfeldt-Jakob disease) in humans through beef consumption. BSE had entered cattle through contaminated feed—sheep offal prepared from sheep with a similar disease called scrapie. Addressing this human health concern, Ferguson predicted in 2002 that between 50 and 150,000 people would die if BSE were to again infect the UK's cattle and sheep, or only up to 50,000 if the disease spared the sheep.[4] The actual human death total was 177. This is greater than 50, so it's in the window. But the forecast is lame for two reasons. First, most of these deaths took place before 2002, so the lower bound is not even a prediction. Second, the range of the window is so broad (the high end is 3,000 times the low end) that it's useless. But Ferguson was wrong in the right direction.

In 2005, Ferguson predicted that up to 200 million people could die from the bird flu. "Around 40 million people died in the 1918 Spanish flu outbreak," he told *The Guardian*.[5] "There are six times more people on the planet now so you could scale it up to around 200 million people probably." As things turned out, 440 people died from the bird flu from 2003 to 2015.[6] In other words, Ferguson's prediction was off by a factor of *nearly 500,000!* But once again, the powers that be didn't hold that against him.

And on that bird-flu miscalculation, Ferguson had stiff competition. David Nabarro, whom the *Guardian* described as "one of the most senior public health experts at the World Health Organisation," said bird flu could kill from 5 to 150 million.[7] An unnamed WHO spokeswoman said "'best case scenario' would be 7.4 million deaths globally." WHO also escaped the error unscathed.

In 2009, Ferguson estimated the mortality rate for swine flu at 0.4 percent. The British government relied on that number to predict a "reasonable worst-case scenario" of 65,000 deaths in the UK. In the end, 457 people died.[8] Ferguson was off by a factor of 142. That's a vast improvement over his bird-flu forecast, but that's not saying much.

IMPERIAL COLLEGE LONDON

The model produced by Imperial College London, which WHO relied on, predicted that the new coronavirus would be about as deadly as the Spanish flu of 1918 (which killed between 18 and 58 million).[9] They predicted the coronavirus would claim 40 million lives worldwide,[10] including 2.2 million in the U.S.,[11] if nothing were done to slow the spread. Forty *million* deaths? Terrifying!

But how were non-experts supposed to check such claims?

Even at the time of that prediction, in late March, the forecast didn't fit the facts. Death rates were already leveling off in some countries, with just over twenty thousand deaths reported worldwide. There were many more deaths to come, of course, but was it really credible that there would be *two thousand times* as many? That seemed hard to swallow.

Something else was fishy. The folks at Imperial College said the coronavirus could cause that many deaths "if left unchecked." But by then lockdowns were already in place in many countries. The prediction almost seemed to be about another world, not the one we were living in. But then champions of the Imperial College model took the mismatch between its predictions and reality as proof of its value. The difference between predicted deaths and actual deaths was to be interpreted as "saved" lives—nearly forty million saved, worldwide.[12]

Many independent scientists used the code from the Imperial College model to run it for other countries. A Ph.D. student at Cornell ran the model for Sweden using actual data from that country, including the kind of voluntary social distancing found in Sweden (where there was no lockdown).[13] The model predicted thousands of deaths per day at the peak. As of July 1, 2020, total deaths attributed to COVID-19 in Sweden had reached about 5,300. The single-day high was 115.[14]

It's absurd for anyone to claim that the model justified lockdowns. This feature—looking good no matter how bad your predictions— reminds us of the classic "Rainmaker Scam." Desperate for rain in the summer of 1894, the people of one Nebraska town hired a "rainmaker" to solve their problem. His "rainmaking" apparatus consisted of "two ten-gallon earthenware crocks," one called the "thundermug," the other the "lightning-mug." They were black boxes to the townspeople, because "as the stuff that does the mischief is inside, the true inward-ness of the contraption is not visible to the naked eye." They had to trust the expert (the rainmaker), who declared that it would rain within five days. Or, if it didn't, that would mean that there was "something wrong with the atmosphere"—for which the rainmaker had a yet more expensive remedy.[15]

That trick of claiming that any outcome proves you were right can really come in handy. One California doctor used it masterfully when the death numbers turned up short. "What we're trying to do is prevent people from dying, that's what we're trying to do in the Bay Area," he said. "The early projections were that there would be 44,000 deaths in the Bay Area. There have been 210 so far so I think we're doing pretty damn good and I certainly don't want to mess with that kind of success."[16]

Even well into the crisis, when other experts had savaged the Imperial College model, authorities and media were still citing it. We expect lockdown champions to keep this up for years. Officials will keep quoting it because it's the only argument they have that they saved millions of people whom the virus would otherwise have killed.

But let's be clear: that use of the model is political, not scientific. There are well-known scientific ways to judge the performance of models. By any of those measures, this early forecast was an abysmal failure.

And yet it inspired the World Health Organization to declare a global emergency. Why? You know the answer. Like Ferguson's earlier epically wrong predictions, it was wrong in the right direction. And politics and the press, not logic or science, decide which direction is right.

WHAT IS A MODEL?

It's not just that the pandemic models happened to be wrong. And it's not just that they were wrong in the right direction—making forecasts that led authorities to believe they could save the world by a massive exercise of government power. The problem was also the way experts used models.

A model is a list of propositions and predictions about an observable phenomenon that we can measure. "Observables" are real things we can see and document, often with instruments—the temperature, or the presence of a virus, or a death.

For instance, consider this very simple model: "The high temperature tomorrow will be the same as today." This model is often wrong, but it can be quite useful. We use that model as a rule-of-thumb for all kinds of decisions—when we're planning what to wear tomorrow, for example.

If anything more important than your clothing choice depends on tomorrow's temperature, you may want to resort to a vastly more complex expert model, using math, physics, statistics, computer code, and current data. Like our simple model above, the expert models incorporate past observations; but even their observations are a lot more complex than just noting that today's high is eighty-five degrees Fahrenheit. They depend on sophisticated ways of gathering data and a sophisticated sense of what data they should and should not include in their calculations.

Models can have two purposes: 1) to explain, or at least to help us understand, how the various "observables" interact, and 2) to make predictions. Some models have one of those aims, some have the other, and some try to do both.

Our rule-of-thumb model doesn't explain the weather. We just use it to guess the temperature tomorrow. A model doesn't need to explain what's happening, or why, to make good or useful guesses about the future.

Indeed, a model could be a perfect predictor but a dismal explainer. Let's say we notice that year by year the U.S. gross domestic product (GDP) is, on average, going up. And we also notice that the number of suicides, too, is increasing annually. A statistical model linking GDP with suicides would make decent *predictions* of the number of suicides. But it wouldn't *explain* the suicides, which are not caused by the increasing prosperity. Rather, both GDP and the number of suicides are going up because the population itself is growing.

And of course, if a model spits out lousy predictions, we can't trust its explanations. Its failure to predict accurately means that it's in error, so we should not believe what it says about how the world works.

Suppose a viral pandemic model includes three propositions: A, B, and C. The model *assumes* each of these statements is true; they are its conceptual inputs. With those in place, numerical inputs can then be used to predict how many people the virus will infect. It says that a million people will be infected by some date. But by that date, in the real world, only ten thousand are infected. Whoops. The model was off by a factor of a hundred. Because the numerical inputs are real-world facts, we now know that something is wrong with A, B, and/or C—with any or all of them.

Our imagined pandemic model has made a huge mistake. How to explain that whopping error? In a perfect world, the experts who created the model, publicized, and used it to create public policy would reassess the assumptions they fed into the model—A, B, and C—find the mistake, and try new ones, which may better match the "observables."

But we don't live in a perfect world with perfect experts. What if experts are loath to admit that they were wrong? (We know that's a real stretch, but stick with us here.) What if they have been feted by the press and promoted to positions of authority and power? They have other options besides the humiliating one of going back to the drawing board. For starters, such experts can stop using the word "predictions" to describe the forecasts that the model has been spitting out. Now they're just "scenarios" or "guidelines" or "projections." But these are just word games. There's little daylight between a forecast, a prediction, a guess, a scenario, and a projection. All those words describe what the model is doing when it says, *If A, B, and C are true, then something like X will happen, give or take a margin of error.* If nothing like X happens, then something's wrong with at least one of the model's conceptual inputs, that is, with one of the propositions that that model assumed to be true. At *least* one of A, B, or C must be wrong.

Our expert model builders still have options. For example, they can claim that their prediction failed because they were a little too shy about one of their insightful propositions. Assumption B, for example, turned out to be even more dramatically true than they had assumed.

Let's say that B was the assumption that the public would obey the expert's advice for mitigation by social distancing, complying with lockdowns, and so forth. Given that input, experts had predicted that there would at some point be between 100,000 and 200,000 total deaths from the new coronavirus in the United States. Or even as many as 240,000, going by the chart on display at the March 31 White House Coronavirus Task Force press conference starring Drs. Anthony Fauci and Deborah Birx.

These numbers were the model's predictions *assuming* B—that is, *given* the public's compliance with the extreme mitigation that the experts were advising. We know this because President Trump explained at that same press conference that the experts had given him a much higher number (2.2 million deaths, in fact) in the case of no mitigation. So as of March 31, the model that the experts were relying on was predicting 100,000 as the smallest possible number of deaths, given full compliance everywhere. "This could be a hell of a bad two weeks," warned the president.[17]

Then, less than two weeks later, the experts changed the forecast. On April 9, Dr. Fauci announced a new predicted total: 60,000 deaths. That was at least 40 percent fewer than he had said just nine days earlier (or 75 percent fewer, taking the upper bound of that prediction): "The final toll currently 'looks more like 60,000 than the 100,000 to 200,000' that U.S. officials previously estimated, Fauci said."[18]

In some places, we know that assumption B was more or less true: people did comply with extreme mitigation. As NPR reported, "The revised analysis [that is, Fauci's new 60,000-death prediction] comes as millions of Americans are living under 'shelter in place' and business shutdown orders that have contributed to massive job losses and other disruptions." The article quoted Fauci himself lauding "the American public's embrace of physical separation and other restrictions."[19] But it wasn't true everywhere. Eight states never locked down, and compliance was patchy even in places with lockdowns.[20]

Fauci's explanation was classic: an expert reluctant to admit error will say he was not wrong. What happened, he will insist, was the real-life B was B-er than the B in the original model. Which is to say that people practiced social distancing even more than the model assumed. According to the NPR report Fauci "also says that the American public's embrace of physical separation and other restrictions is sharply reducing projections of the death toll from the respiratory virus." Recall that the one hundred thousand total deaths Fauci had predicted just nine days earlier was the *best*-case scenario, based on the maximum mitigation.

With less mitigation, the experts had claimed there could be as many as 240,000 dead; and with no mitigation, 2.2 million would have died. So, it was nonsense for Dr. Fauci to say, nine days later, that "the American public's embrace of physical separation and other restrictions" was "sharply reducing" the model's predictions. In fact, their maximum embrace of those mitigations had been baked into the model. The facts on the ground hadn't *modified* the model's predictions.

THE FALSE PROMISE OF MODELS

If you forget everything else about models, remember this: you can't get out of a model what you didn't put in. This goes for simple models and complicated ones. Models only say what we tell them to say.

Suppose a scientist has been using our simple temperature model that predicts tomorrow will probably have the same high temperature as today. She notices it does a pretty good job. So she writes a peer-reviewed science paper explaining just how well it did. A journalist sees the paper and writes a story, "Scientist Discovers Yesterday's High Temperature Linked to Today's High Temperature."

In fact, she discovered no such thing. She assumed it from the beginning! She didn't discover anything new. She told the model what to say.

The same thing is true for any model. Modelers want specific results, and so they build their models to spit out those results.

Here's a typical example. A May 12, 2020, headline from a local CBS affiliate in Minnesota announced, "An updated model from the University of Minnesota and state's health department is predicting that COVID-19 cases will peak in late-July with 25,000 deaths possible—if the stay-at-home order is extended until the end of May."[21] As of that date, daily deaths were in the upper teens and low twenties, with 614 total deaths in the state. And yet local journalists were taking seriously a model that predicted twenty-five *thousand* deaths.

Minnesota's governor, Tim Walz, said the modeling showed that "if you social distance you buy more time."[22] The governor was wrong. The success of social distancing was an *input* to the model. Models don't prove social distancing works—they *assume* it. The success of social distancing isn't anything models even could discover. Indeed, it may not even be true! True or not, this was an assumption baked into them from the start.[23]

How did things play out in Minnesota? By July 1, the total deaths reported were 1,458. The daily rate of new deaths was in the low single digits, and trending toward 0.

"A Buggy Mess"

We finally turn to the Imperial College model built by their "COVID-19 Response" team, with lead author Neil M. Ferguson, whom we have already met.[24] This model attempts to predict not just infection rates, case numbers, and deaths, but also how human beings will behave. It tries to simulate, for example, the supply and use of hospital resources. According to a *Nature* report,[25] this model was "based around trying to understand how people move between three main states, and how quickly: individuals are either susceptible (S) to the virus; have become infected (I); and then either recover (R) or die." It belongs to an ambitious class of models that "subdivide people into smaller groups—by age, sex, health status, employment, number of contacts, and so on—to set who meets whom, when and in which places."

Finally, "Using detailed information on population size and density, how old people are, transport links, the size of social networks and health-care provision, modelers build a virtual copy of a city, region or an entire country using differential equations to govern the movements and interactions of population groups in space and time."

The *Nature* article pointed out, though, that "as the groups are broken into smaller, more representative social subsets to better reflect reality, the models get increasingly complicated."

And what about unknown factors? "Some parameters, meanwhile, must be entirely assumed," the article admits. "The Imperial team had to surmise, for instance, that there is no natural immunity to COVID-19—so the entire population starts out in the susceptible group—and that people who recover from COVID-19 are immune to reinfection in the short term."

So we have assumptions and simplifications galore. Some are no better than guesses. And this is how the model "estimated 2.2 million US deaths."

These models are hideously complex. This one was so complex, in fact, that it didn't work when it was independently tested two months after its release. A veteran software engineer investigated the model code and found it riddled with bugs. So much so that the model gave "very different results given identical inputs."[26] The differences weren't small.

Recall that models can only say what they're told to say. According to the software engineer who found the bugs in this one, the problem was that R_e, the effective rate of infection, was "both an input to *and an output* of these models and is routinely adjusted for different environments and situations. Models that consume their own outputs as inputs…can lead to rapid divergence and incorrect prediction."[27]

The story gets even stranger. The model the Imperial College Team finally released wasn't the one they had used for their famous forecast, but a modified version. The code they released on GitHub (a popular code-sharing site) was "a heavily modified derivative of" the original code, "after having been upgraded for over a month by a team from Microsoft and others." The software engineer concluded, "Clearly, Imperial are too embarrassed by the state of it ever to release it of their own free will, which is unacceptable given that it was paid for by the taxpayer and belongs to them." The *Nature* paper also quoted Ferguson saying the model "code was not released when his team's projections on the coronavirus pandemic were first made public, but the team is working with Microsoft to tidy up the code and make it available."[28] Wow. How could code that wasn't fit for public viewing be fit for making decisions affecting billions of people?

Two other engineers, writing for the *Telegraph*, said they were "profoundly disturbed at what we discovered. The model appears to be totally unreliable" and it "could go down in history as the most devastating software mistake of all time, in terms of economic costs and lives lost." They noted that the model seemed to have been written in the highly antiquated programming language Fortran. Why is that a problem? The language "contains inherent problems with its grammar and the way it assigns values, which can give way to multiple design flaws and numerical inaccuracies. One file in the Imperial model contained 15,000 lines of code."[29]

It was, the engineers concluded, a "buggy mess that looks more like a bowl of angel hair pasta than a finely tuned piece of programming."[30]

Alas, no one knew this on March 15, 2020, when Imperial College first made public their results, along with two advised "strategies."

The two strategies recommended for Great Britain were: "a) mitigation, which focuses on slowing but not necessarily stopping epidemic spread—reducing peak healthcare demand while protecting those most at risk of severe disease from infection, and b) suppression, which aims to reverse epidemic growth, reducing case numbers to low levels and maintaining that situation indefinitely."

According to the Imperial College, "*optimal* mitigation policies...*might* reduce peak healthcare demand by ⅔ and deaths by half. However, the resulting mitigated epidemic would still likely result in hundreds of thousands of deaths and health systems...being overwhelmed many times over" (emphasis added). By mitigation they meant such things as, in their own words:

- combining home isolation of suspect cases
- home quarantine of those living in the same household as suspect cases
- and social distancing of the elderly and others at most risk of severe disease

But the team advised suppression over mitigation. That meant a combination of—again, in their words:

- social distancing of the entire population
- home isolation of cases and household quarantine of their family members
- school and university closures
- and other such policies, many of which were adopted

Authorities would need to enforce suppression, they said, for "potentially 18 months or more," until a vaccine could be discovered.

What if society just mitigated? It would be a catastrophe. "In the most effective mitigation strategy examined, which leads to a single, relatively short epidemic," they wrote, "even if all patients were able to be treated, we predict there would still be in the order of 250,000 deaths in GB [Great Britain], and 1.1–1.2 million in the US."

Okay. But with suppression, if authorities acted quickly, deaths in Great Britain could be much lower, between fifty-six hundred to forty-eight thousand, depending on how the disease was transmitted and the use of ICUs. They said numbers would be proportional for the U.S., but did not give any figures.[31]

Almost a month later, on April 13, total deaths in the United Kingdom were 11,329. Since that's on the low end of the range assuming suppression, does that mean the model was right? No.

Much of the world did end up adopting the "suppression" measures that the Imperial College recommended (and more)—"social distancing," closing schools, and a lockdown that quarantined not only the sick but even the healthy. But there's no proof that the lockdowns did much to "flatten the curve," slow the spread of the disease, or change the course of the pandemic—as we'll show in detail in chapter 9. For now, suffice it to say that the infection and death curves in countries and U.S. states seemed indifferent to government lockdowns.

In any case, the business-as-usual predictions were always way too high to be believed.

The Imperial College model had predicted that with no mitigation about 510,000 would die in Great Britain and 2.2 million in the United States. These are staggering numbers. There are about 66.7 million people in the UK and 328.2 million in the United States. The model predicted that deaths per day per 100,000 people would peak at about 21 in Britain (around June 1) and 17 in the United States (around June 20).[32]

That translates into about fourteen thousand deaths per day in the UK and fifty-six thousand per day in the United States! We're shocked that anybody believed these astounding numbers.

Of course, there is no real way to measure whether the model got these morbid predictions right. We can't compare what did happen (both countries suppressed and mitigated) with the counterfactual world where it didn't happen (if they hadn't). Anyway, the no-mitigation numbers are so large that anyone not invested in the model should have doubted them out of the gate.

The model predicted 670 per 100,000 dead of coronavirus with no mitigation. Compare that to the horrific Spanish flu of 1918. It befell a world with poor medical care at the end of a global war. Between 17 and 58 million were killed worldwide.[33] The CDC estimates that about 675,000 Americans died, out of a U.S. population of about 106 million.[34]

That was 637 dead per 100,000—*fewer* than Imperial College was predicting for the coronavirus without mitigation. The model was therefore predicting that even with modern medicine, coronavirus would be deadlier than the Spanish flu. Even without knowing the sorry state of the model code, keen observers should have been suspicious.

THE IHME MODEL

Another official model that played a big role in the response to the virus in the United States was the one produced by the Institute for Health Metrics and Evaluation (IHME) at the University of Washington.[35] This model was like the Imperial College model in that it purported to say something not just about how many people the virus would infect, but how many ICU beds they would need. It even revealed, Magic-8-Ball style, how many hospital admissions there would be, and how many ventilators would be needed in each *state*. Its minders updated the model regularly, using the latest statistics.

In its favor, the IHME not only gave the expected number for each of these metrics; they also provided plus-or-minus bounds for each. That is, they admitted that the model wasn't precise. Only the bounds they gave were often so wide as to make the predictions meaningless. For example, on April 13, 2020, the model predicted that the United States would need 59,600 hospital beds to cope with coronavirus on April 14. This prediction came with uncertainty bounds of 13,000 and 192,000. That's a huge range, considering it was just trying to divine what would happen the next day!

The same model run predicted there would be 1,953 reported deaths on April 14, with a range of 292 to 6,771. There were, in fact, 2,299 deaths reported on that day. Again, this prediction was for one day ahead.[36]

It's odd that the uncertainty bounds would be that large for a twenty-four-hour forecast. This should have been a dead giveaway not to trust the model too much. Oddly, neither the experts nor the political decision makers ever drew that conclusion.

Strangely, the model was more precise for forecasts two weeks out, than for predictions about tomorrow. This bizarre feature showed up every time the model was run. The earliest prediction from IHME's model, on March 25, was that there would be 2,341 reported deaths on April 14, with an uncertainty window of 1,149 to 4,844. Thus, the actual number for April 14 (2,299) was predicted considerably better on March 25 than on April 13.

Like all models, the IHME one was imperfect, but it got some things right. In truth, it's easier to bat .400 than it is to create a pandemic epidemiological model that nails all of its predictions. The real problem, as we will see below, is that so many people naively think perfect models for complex behavior even exist.

Political advisors took worst-case scenarios from highly uncertain models as if they were perfect. In the wrong hands, rough-and-ready tools became weapons of mass destruction.

HIGH SCHOOL SCIENCE FAIR

Perhaps the weirdest fact about coronavirus models was described in a *New York Times* article, "The Untold Story of the Birth of Social Distancing." The idea started as "an important discovery kicked off by a high school research project pursued by the daughter of a scientist at the Sandia National Laboratories."

In 2006, fourteen-year-old Laura Glass developed a model of social networks in her high school in Albuquerque. That's impressive. But what's troubling is that this science-fair project gave rise to the template for shutting the world down on the signal from health authorities.

This dystopian progression started when Laura's dad, Sandia National Laboratories scientist David Glass, took notice. The two expanded on the idea by applying the model to a pandemic, and they published a paper on it with two other authors in a CDC journal. It's called "Targeted Social Distancing Designs for Pandemic Influenza." [37]

The abstract summarizing the paper explains, "For influenza as infectious as 1957–1958 Asian flu ($\approx$50 percent infected), closing schools and keeping children and teenagers at home reduced the attack rate by >90%." Notice the tone. It suggests—no, it *proclaims*—that closing schools works.

This sounds like the paper's authors were describing real school closures. But they weren't. Schools were closed only in a simulation.

What really happened was this: the authors of the paper told the model to say the attack rate would be lower and, behold, it was.

The excited authors of this paper sent their simulation to a Dr. D. A. Henderson, who was, as the *New York Times* explains, "the leader of the international effort to eradicate smallpox and had been named by [President] Bush to help oversee the nation's biodefense efforts after the 2001 terrorist attacks."

Henderson pushed back, saying that "it made no sense to force schools to close or public gatherings to stop." Indeed, if authorities adopted such policies, he rightly discerned, the result would be "significant disruption of the social functioning of communities" and "possibly serious economic problems." Henderson had vast scientific expertise and broad and pertinent experience dealing with such crises. His advice? We should "tough it out: Let the pandemic spread, treat people who get sick and work quickly to develop a vaccine to prevent it from coming back."[38]

The CDC didn't know what to do if and when a pandemic should hit. Go with Henderson's plan, which had always worked before and would likely work again, or go with the simulation? So, in 2008 the agency put out a survey of the U.S. adult population.[39] Here's what the survey revealed, according to the abstract:

> Survey results suggest that if community mitigation measures are instituted, most respondents would comply with recommendations but would be challenged to do so if their income or job were severely compromised. The results also indicate that community mitigation measures could cause problems for persons with lower incomes and for racial and ethnic minorities. Twenty-four percent of respondents said that they would not have anyone available to take care of them if they became sick with pandemic influenza. Given these results, planning and public engagement will be needed to encourage the public to be prepared.

In other words, the CDC found that lockdowns would cause big problems. Why did it support them, then? Well, it also did a second survey.

This time it sampled not just ordinary citizens but "representatives from the organized stakeholder public."[40] These elite "stakeholder representatives from affected sectors of the population expressed a high level of support for the…proposed package of control measures." And in group sessions, the citizens came around to agreeing. The proposed measures would require sick people—and people who knew the sick people—to stay home. The proposed lockdown would mean "canceling large public gatherings and altering work patterns to keep people apart" and also "closing schools and large day care facilities for an extended period."

And the "administration ultimately sided with the proponents of social distancing and shutdowns," the *New York Times* explained, "though their victory was little noticed outside of public health circles. Their policy would become the basis for government planning and would be used extensively in simulations used to prepare for pandemics."[41] So, a survey steered by people with a vested interest in political control led the government to set aside Henderson's tried-and-true scientific expertise and experience.

And that's how, a decade before anyone had heard of the novel coronavirus, the public health bureaucracy of the United States government committed itself and its citizens to an unprecedented experiment. The plan they put in place called for drastic measures that they knew—because their own research had told them—could cripple the economy, severely harm disadvantaged Americans, and subject millions of people to health risks from the response itself.

Then, in 2020, the government finally got to play the game with live ammo. All because a high school kid had told a computer what to say.

IF THE MODEL MAKES BAD PREDICTIONS, REJECT IT

When the government-favored models started to come up short, some defended them. One excuse was to say the models were never meant to be good. Really.

Scott Adams, the creator of *Dilbert*, is a keen cultural critic who isn't afraid to swim against the tide. Still, he fell under the spell of models early on and had a hard time snapping out of it. "Prediction models are not designed to be accurate," he said, when the gap between the models and facts became obvious.[42] "They are designed to be useful. If you don't understand that distinction, nothing you say about the models moves the ball forward."

That's false. Accuracy about predictions is exactly what the models are for. That's why we call them predictive models.

One of Adams's follow-up claims was even worse. "Prediction models are built to persuade the public toward expert consensus," he tweeted. "They are not snapshots of the future. Debating the accuracy of models misses the point of them." He seemed to be saying that models are an expert *conspiracy*. First, the experts come to some sort of consensus—who knows how, perhaps through augury. Then they build a fancy model that will trick the great unwashed into buying what the experts have already decided.

When it comes to technocratic experts wandering outside their domain, we're skeptical. But not as cynical as Adams. Adams would have us believe that the modelers and their heralds know their models are wrong and cooked them up to control us.

We think most experts believe they're telling the truth. They've just put far too much trust in their mental castles.

We know that if a model makes lousy forecasts, at least some of its statements must be wrong. (There are ways to figure this out; but, unfortunately, only long after the model has run.) That is, it must misrepresent reality. If planners act based on that model's flawed forecasts, they're making a mistake.

If a model can't explain reality, no one should use it for planning.

In fact, even if a model *seems* to explain reality, we should still be cautious. A model can sometimes make accurate predictions in error.

Remember the statistical model that predicts suicide numbers from GDP: if GDP increases, suicides will likely increase. And they do! The model nailed it! But only because both GDP and suicides increase with population size. A planner would be a fool to use this statistical model to say, *Let's lower the GDP. That way we can lower suicides.*

No.

At a *minimum*, before we let any model guide our choices, we must insist that it prove it can make pretty accurate predictions.

And how can it do that? It has to do one simple thing: make accurate predictions of data it has never seen before. This is so simple; it's hard to believe that models are rarely subjected to this test. But they almost never are. At best, a smart modeler will tweak a model to fit the details of, say, a past viral outbreak, until it does a pretty good job of "predicting" old outcomes—that is, of reproducing what we already know.

That would be okay, except at this stage model creators too often convince themselves that the model has proved itself. In fact, all they know is that if they tweak the model using the numbers they know, then the model can reproduce those known numbers. To really prove itself, the model instead must be able to predict future data—data that neither the model nor the modelers have seen before—accurately. Only then does it make sense to use the model to make predictions. Otherwise, there's no good reason to trust what it predicts, let alone to use it to guide national or international policy.

Now in the coronavirus case, the IHME model, the Imperial College model, and others were new, and not yet tested on COVID data. How could they have been, since the bug itself was new?

And yet the models' creators would argue their models weren't new at all. They were just extensions of prior epidemiological models, tuned to current research. The Imperial College COVID model, for example, pointed to older models.[43] This is standard for scientific work, which always builds on earlier work.

But that didn't guarantee that the new coronavirus model would be any good. That would depend on, among other factors, how closely the prior research fit the new facts—something there was no way to know at the start of an outbreak.

That doesn't mean we can't use models for guidance. But this vast lack of certainty means we should not trust the model out of the gate. We should attach healthy, if unquantifiable, uncertainty to the claims of any model, especially when it is first used.

USE WHAT WE HAVE, NOT WHAT WE DON'T HAVE

Doubting the unproven models doesn't leave us high and dry. We still have simpler models that have survived the tests of time and proven themselves by making accurate predictions in the past. Such tried-and-true models do not pretend to predict the course of a new disease with precision. But their predictions are likely to be in the ballpark. We can marry them with what we know from other sources. For example, suppose a homely statistical model predicted, *given the past history of viruses that seem to be like this one, we expect that X number of people will die in this one.* Hospitals could use that information, along with copious experience from annual flu seasons, to better allocate resources. And as the outbreak progresses, the assumptions should be adjusted. Maybe what we thought was like the Spanish flu virus of 1918 turns out to be more like the swine flu virus of 2009.

Any complex, real-world decision will involve assumptions, guesses, and analogies. The problem arises when we think we have a perfect oracle, grounded in the eternal truths of math or the constants of physics. Even physicists rarely enjoy certainty. Yes, they can model with wondrous accuracy how a single electron wends its way through a known magnetic field—but there are fewer *simpler* processes than that. And that's physics! Pretending that we can predict just what will happen to seven-plus billion people in a pandemic in anything but gross statistical terms is beyond wishful thinking. It's delusional. And, as we've seen, it can be deadly.

Expecting such unattainable accuracy drives the incentive to supply it, much as expecting accurate astrology encourages hucksters to provide detailed horoscopes. We need to dry up this market for the impossible—at least among the class that makes the rules we have to obey. If we don't, it will continue to leave death and destruction in its wake.

CHAPTER 8

WHY DID WE BELIEVE LOCKDOWNS WOULD WORK?

Extraordinary claims require extraordinary evidence.

—*Carl Sagan[1]*

On April 18, conservative columnist Rich Lowry spoke for many when he argued against lockdown skeptics: "If we are going to have 60,000 deaths with people not leaving their homes for more than a month, the number of deaths obviously would have been higher—much higher—if everyone had gone about business as usual. We didn't lock down the country to try to *prevent* 60,000 deaths; we locked down the country to *limit* deaths to 60,000 (or whatever the ultimate toll is)."[2]

Lowry was expressing what seemed to be common sense: however many people died with the lockdowns, the deaths would have been far worse without them. As late as May 8, Gallup reported that 87 percent of Americans were either "very" or "moderately confident" that social distancing had saved lives.[3] In fact, Pew reported around the same time, 68 percent of Americans were worried that states would be too quick to lift restrictions.[4] A partisan divide was opening—with more Republicans than Democrats skeptical of both the lockdowns and the media coverage. But if we believe the polls, most Americans were still more scared of the virus than of the lockdowns. After all, flimsy as its basis in fact or science was, the number that stuck in everyone's heads was 2.2 million deaths—as predicted by the Imperial College London model and endorsed by WHO.

As we've seen, the original case for the lockdown was to "flatten the curve"—to keep the number of cases of COVID-19 from overwhelming the healthcare system. It was supposed to last a couple of weeks.[5] But it soon become clear that, with a few exceptions, hospitals in the United States would not be overwhelmed by coronavirus cases. In fact, the glut of empty hospital beds became something of an embarrassment. Google and other search engines did their best to bury these stories, but you can still find them if you scroll long enough.[6]

At that point, authorities pivoted to a *different* excuse: the lockdown would save lives by preventing infections. And with that change, any clear end date for the restrictions on our movement and basic rights disappeared. The new reasoning was that our costly measures were saving lives not by spreading out the high number of cases to lower the peak but by *reducing* that number. The rampant spread of the virus, which the authorities had described as inevitable just a couple of weeks earlier, was now the thing to avoid. Most people, including Rich Lowry, took this revised justification for the lockdown to heart. It's why we were still sheltering in place in May.

Most of us relied on what seemed like logic and common sense. If the coronavirus was spread to other people by coughing, sneezing, licking our fingers, touching doorknobs, and the like, then whatever we did to reduce those infection-spreading actions would help. At one extreme are clueless people packed sardine-like in a subway car. They're hacking and coughing and wiping their snotty hands on the railings while sharing snacks for forty-five minutes every day as they ride from Flatbush Ave. in Brooklyn to Central Park North, never bothering to wash their hands or cough into their elbows. At the other end are hermits spread out across the South Dakota prairie, each wearing a hazmat suit and avoiding others like the plague.

We don't need a multi-million-dollar study to guess how the coronavirus will fare in these two scenarios. The misanthropic hermit with the hazmat suit hunkered down in the Badlands need not worry about coming down with COVID-19. The carefree lawyer with bad hygiene riding the subway to get to his job in Manhattan is at risk.

But those are the extremes. Reality is somewhere in the middle, with or without mandated lockdowns. And we had plenty of options between "business as usual" and ordering 95 percent of the public to stay at home. So, we still have to ask: First, did we have good reason, even at the start, to think that lockdowns *as actually practiced* would save millions of lives? And second, with the benefit of hindsight, do we have good reason to think they did?

We'll tackle that first question here, and the second in chapter 9.

How Pandemics Begin and End

Let's begin with a quick overview of basic epidemiology. Fortunately, if you followed the news at all in 2020, you've already seen most of what you need to know.

Think of a viral epidemic or pandemic from the viewpoint of the virus. To the virus, every susceptible human is a chance to cause another infection. Before a victim even knows that she is coming down with something, a respiratory virus has multiplied in her upper respiratory tract, which is now shedding thousands of tiny virus particles.

Mucus is their FedEx. Hand delivery is one good option—which is why we shifted from handshakes to fist bumps in 2020. But airmail works too. The big jumbo jets are visible droplets, which can fly short distances in close quarters. The tiny carriers are microscopic droplets, which can hang in the air for many minutes, or aerosols, which, because they are even tinier, can hang for hours.

Think of the person infected with coronavirus as a virus distribution center sending unwanted packages to unwitting recipients.

R_e is the average number of successful deliveries from one of these centers. That number doesn't have to be high for the virus to cause a huge outbreak. In fact, R_e just needs to be greater than one, which means the virus is infecting more than one new person from each infected person, on average. When that happens, the outbreak will grow *exponentially*. That is, the number of infected people will double at regular intervals—every day, or every three days, or every week. When R_e is *less* than one, in contrast, then the number of infected people will drop by half at regular intervals.

The good news is that at some point R_e does fall below one. One way this happens is *herd immunity*. People survive viral infections when their bodies mount a successful immune response. In a remarkable process, our bodies experiment with antibodies until they find the right one to conquer the virus. That successful antibody then lingers in the body for years, ready to shut the virus down if it encounters it again. This is how people who recover from a virus become immune to a repeat infection.

As more and more infected people recover, it becomes harder for the virus to be passed on. There may be some distribution centers still shipping the unwanted packages, but fewer addresses will accept them. At some point, the number of successful deliveries per center falls below one, and the end of the outbreak is in sight. This is how almost all viral outbreaks come and go.

A vaccine can speed up herd immunity by exposing lots of people to a harmless version of a virus (sometimes just a part of it). This allows their bodies to create the antibody without ever really being infected.

But it takes time for researchers to develop and test vaccines. So vaccines aren't usually a solution for new viruses. Natural herd immunity comes much sooner.

In theory, we could also reduce R_e by changing our behavior. That is, we could use what we know about how the virus spreads to impede it. In effect, we'd block the delivery routes between distribution centers and recipients. This is the idea behind social distancing.

If communities can change their behavior to hinder viral spread, then this would reduce R_e.

As simple as this seems, it's hard to show that it works. Just because we *intend* to lower R_e doesn't mean we'll succeed. After all, viruses don't care about our good intentions.

WHO KNEW

Were authorities right to believe that if they closed schools and businesses, issued stay-at-home orders, mandated face coverings, and compelled us to stand six feet apart at the checkout lines, it would cut off those delivery routes and save many lives? Were we right to believe them?

Perhaps the most surprising witness for the prosecution is…the World Health Organization itself. Though it received little attention, WHO issued a report as recently as October 2019 on "non-pharmaceutical public health measures" in fighting a flu pandemic. The executive summary said the evidence in favor of these measures was "limited."[7] Based on the rest of the report, that was an understatement.

The non-drug-based interventions WHO considered were "personal protective measures (e.g. hand hygiene, respiratory etiquette and face masks)," "environmental measures" (cleaning and disinfecting), "social distancing measures (e.g. contact tracing, isolation of sick individuals, quarantine of exposed individuals, school measures and closures, workplace measures and closures, and avoiding crowding)," and "travel-related measures (e.g. travel advice, entry and exit screening, internal travel restrictions and border closure)."

In other words, the lockdowns. Almost everyone assumed they would work. WHO, in contrast, concluded: not so much.

Hand washing makes sense, but studies haven't shown that it works. Controlled trials "have not found that hand hygiene is effective in reducing transmission of laboratory-confirmed influenza." Still, it's easy to do.

Face masks also make sense, though they're much more of a hassle. Again, though, when it comes to people without symptoms wearing them in public, "there is no evidence that this is effective in reducing transmission."

Perhaps most controversially, WHO reported, "Travel-related measures are unlikely to be successful in most locations because current screening tools such as thermal scanners cannot identify pre-symptomatic infections and afebrile infections, and travel restrictions and travel bans are likely to have prohibitive economic consequences."

They also warned that "social distancing measures (for example, contact tracing, isolation, quarantine, school and workplace measures and closures, and avoiding crowding) can be highly disruptive, and the cost of these measures must be weighed against their potential impact." Moreover, they may do less than most people assume. They judged the quality of evidence supporting the value of these measures to be "very low."

Lockdowns, they said, can even spread disease, since "household quarantine can increase the risks of household members becoming infected." Compliance is always a problem, and herding healthy and at-risk people together might just spread the virus to at-risk people. "Workplace closure," they cautioned, "should be a last step that is only considered in extraordinarily severe epidemics and pandemics."

How bad is "extraordinarily severe"? Thanks to the work of the CDC,[8] we don't have to guess. Their chart (Figure 8.1) shows that only one flu pandemic in over a hundred years has qualified: the 1918 Spanish flu pandemic.

So, even the official wisdom on pandemics warned of the high cost of extreme social distancing. That same wisdom acknowledged that studies of these measures had never proved that they work, and in many cases had suggested they don't (a point we'll unpack next).

Why didn't this bombshell of a report make headlines around the world? It came out just a few months before the coronavirus panic. It was sober and thorough, containing references to over 240 scientific papers and other works.

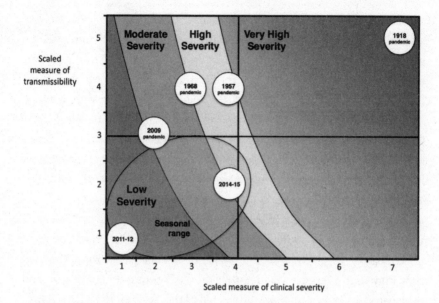

Figure 8.1. The Pandemic Severity Assessment Framework, in chart form, from the *Centers for Disease Control and Prevention* the endnote number).[9]

But few people wanted calm reasoning when the panic set in. Once the pandemic escalated from a medical thing to a political and social thing, the report seemed dull. Instead, WHO, the CDC,[10] and everyone else urged us to be the guinea pigs in a multi-trillion-dollar social experiment that had never been run before, and with precious little evidence in its favor.

WHAT WORKS?

The WHO report focused on flu transmission. That makes sense, because influenza has been a bigger threat than previous coronaviruses. A Google Scholar search for articles in science and medical journals with the word *influenza* returns 1.4 million hits from 1970 to 2019. Changing the word to *coronavirus* drops the hits by more than 90 percent.

That's okay, though. We want to know how respiratory viruses spread through the population, and the two classes of virus are a lot alike on that score. As WHO put it, "COVID-19 and influenza viruses have a similar disease presentation."[11] Both are membrane-wrapped RNA viruses around a tenth of a micron across. Both infect the linings of our upper and lower respiratory tracts, causing similar symptoms in most cases. So, it's reasonable to think they would be passed in similar ways.

Unfortunately, even our knowledge of flu transmission is limited. As one article from 2019 explains, "Despite extensive clinical experience and decades of research on influenza, it is still not fully understood how influenza is transmitted among humans."[12] How can this be, with over a million papers?

The answer is in that phrase "among humans." We're complicated. Just think of what you do on a normal day—when you're not quarantined. You drive, shop, type, eat, touch the gas nozzle at the filling station, and your phone, and the handle on the community coffee pot, and the restroom door, and your phone again, and after all that—your *face*, maybe twenty times every hour.[13] Think of all the things you do with and around other people.

Now, let's say you want to test how sneezing into the elbow compares to sneezing into the hands. We think elbow sneezing will hinder flu transmission. That's the hypothesis. The gold standard for testing this would be a perfectly controlled experiment on two groups that are the same except for their method of sneezing. But how on earth would you set up such an experiment on people in real life, none of whom are identical?

So we go for bronze instead, settling for three imperfect kinds of studies:

1. Contrived studies with a handful of volunteers
2. Simplistic computer models
3. Limited observations of real situations (no control)

Conclusions from the first two kinds of studies are hard to trust because they lack realism. The third kind of study doesn't lend itself to general conclusions. Scientists refer to the third kind of evidence as *anecdotal*. That means that it's more like storytelling than like rigorous science.

When your uncle Ted swears that chewing ginger root cures migraines, he's giving you anecdotal evidence. The problem is not that he has no evidence, but rather that he's generalizing from the experience (and the strong belief) of one person. So, his claim isn't convincing. Likewise, if it were reported that there were 4.3 percent fewer flu cases in a culture where elbow-sneezing is the norm, that wouldn't be very compelling. There would be several ways to interpret the data. Any number of other cultural differences could be the real explanation for the lower incidence of the flu.

Of course, just because we don't have a controlled study on elbow-sneezing doesn't mean it's worthless. It might work. Besides, it seems better, which is enough support for the idea since it's so easy to do.

We can't justify every mitigation that way, though. Some other measures come with severe costs in terms of lives and wellbeing. We knew from the outset that closing businesses and issuing shelter-in-place orders would cut to the quick. It was one thing for officials to inform the public about the virus, urge low-cost precautions, and advise us to do what we could. It was another thing for state and local governments to terrify the public and then impose risky, high-cost measures on almost everyone—measures that, as it happens, lack solid evidence to commend them.

THE SKETCHY SCIENCE OF SOCIAL DISTANCING

Take the six-foot rule. It's common sense that the farther apart people are—remember our imaginary hermits in hazmat suits in South Dakota—the less likely they are to pass an infection to each other. The coronavirus seemed especially deadly in many places with high population density, such as New York City. But what's so special about six feet? As it turns out, not that much.

Experts agree that we can pass the flu virus either by contact (as when snotty hands touch a handrail, which is touched by other hands) or by droplets (spray from a cough) or by aerosol (microscopic mist from coughs, sneezes, or speech). We know that aerosol particles can stay suspended in air for hours,[14] and small droplets for minutes.[15] Yet for years public health officials have downplayed airborne transmission. A WHO document, for instance, describes how larger droplets are "assumed to be the main mode of transmission for influenza." That's a key assumption, since the six-foot separation rule hinges on it.[16] Six feet has merit for avoiding big droplets, but it provides a false security if smaller droplets and aerosols play a large role in transmitting a virus, as many studies have indicated.[17]

That applies to the coronavirus as much as to the flu. A study published during the pandemic showed that the new coronavirus, like the earlier SARS-CoV-1, hangs in the air for over an hour in aerosol form.[18]

Even for protection against large droplets, the recommended distance varies. WHO said 1 meter, or about 3 feet, a number the CDC agreed with because of SARS research.[19] Taiwan went with 1.5 meters.[20] A U.S. Army colonel and chief of Preventive Medicine Services, Public Health Command Europe, said, "I recommend you stay 12 feet apart."[21] Some scientists in the UK complained that the two-meter rule (about 6.5 feet) adopted there was based on "very fragile evidence."[22]

So the six-foot rule is cold comfort. If you walk through a grocery aisle where an infected person was speaking a minute or two earlier, you'll probably inhale small droplets or aerosol particles from that person. Outdoors, where even a gentle breeze quickly sweeps aerosols away, your odds are much better. That fits with a recent report that coronavirus transmission to multiple people almost always happens indoors.[23]

WHAT ABOUT MASKS?

The story of masks in the coronavirus episode is byzantine. They weren't part of the national lockdowns, but many cities, counties, and states started mandating face coverings in April.

At first, neither WHO nor the CDC encouraged masks for healthy people, perhaps because it's so easy to misuse them and they feared shortages among healthcare workers. Moreover, the WHO report we referred to above says, "There is a moderate overall quality of evidence that face masks do not have a substantial effect on transmission of influenza."[24] They based that conclusion on the results of ten randomized controlled trials. Still, WHO judged that masks were worth using in severe pandemics because of "mechanistic plausibility."

The messaging from WHO and the CDC did not inspire confidence. They seemed to be saying both that masks don't work, and that people shouldn't hoard them because healthcare workers need them. Surgeon General Jerome Adams managed to distill this confusing message into a single tweet. On February 28, he wrote, "Seriously people-STOP BUYING MASKS! They are NOT effective in preventing general public from catching #Coronavirus, but if healthcare providers can't get them to care for sick patients, it puts them and our communities at risk!" This defied common sense: Masks work for healthcare workers but not for the general public? It looked like the CDC was trying to herd sheep rather than reason with adults. Perhaps the public could detect that, since many wore masks anyway, even before cities and states started mandating them. When the CDC changed its tune in April, it created even more suspicion.[25]

Part of the appeal of surgical masks may be that, like N95 respirators, they look more serious than bandanas. But surgical masks and N95s are quite different. The former are soft and loose-fitting, while respirators are stiff and tight-fitting. They also serve different purposes. "Surgical masks," as one study notes, "are primarily designed to protect the environment from the wearer, whereas the respirators are supposed to protect the wearer from the environment."[26] Surgeons wear masks during surgery to protect others from spit and droplets. We presume that they could do the same for non-surgeons.

Healthcare workers use fit-tested N95 respirators, not surgical masks, when working with infectious patients. Unlike the other options, an N95 respirator can prevent you from inhaling 95 percent of the tiny virus-carrying particles that otherwise would have entered

your respiratory system. Like the others, it will also catch larger droplets. Beyond that, it can reduce the spread of the particles from your
mouth and nose (unless it has a valve).

But it has to be properly fitted to work. If there's a gap, contaminated air can stream right through it, taking the path of least resistance.
Fit around the nose bridge is tricky. Facial hair is a no-no. A proper fit
comes with a trade-off, too: it makes breathing a chore. That can make
this or any mask risky for small children, or anyone else who has a hard
time breathing.[27]

Even in this best-case scenario, it's unclear how much the average
wearer would reduce the chances of infection.[28] And in any case, mask
mandates in the United States didn't recommend this best-case scenario.
As of April 20, only a handful of U.S. states required face coverings in
public.[29] Local authorities, in Los Angeles County and Washington,
D.C., for example, had issued most of those mandates[30]—which often
required the general public to wear cloth coverings *instead of* surgical
and N95 masks to prevent shortages for healthcare workers. Authorities
admitted that cloth coverings would offer wearers little protection but
claimed they might protect others by catching large droplets from
infected users.[31] From what we saw in L.A. and Washington, D.C., most
people did wear face coverings indoors when they were required to, but
usually these were just cloth or surgical masks. N95 use was rare.

We don't know whether cloth face-coverings do much good in real
use. We do know that there is no strong evidence that they do. And there
is evidence that they could do more harm than good in some cases. For
one thing, they're easy to contaminate. And if mask wearers think they're
protected, they may spend more time closer to other people, including sick
people. Economists call risk-offsetting behavior like this the Peltzman
Effect, after the economist who first described it.

In the end, face coverings may have been as much about signaling
and social control as about science and safety.

CHAPTER 9

DID THE LOCKDOWNS WORK?

We are ready to accept almost any explanation of the present crisis of our civilization except one: that the present state of the world may be the result of genuine error on our own part and that the pursuit of some of our most cherished ideals has apparently produced results utterly different from those which we expected.

—F. A. Hayek[1]

W e have argued that the scientific basis for thinking we could save millions of lives through mandatory social distancing and lockdowns was flimsy. But the experiment went ahead anyway, for better or for worse. Did the lockdowns do what was advertised?

The first warning signs came in April. Officials had predicted a huge surge in COVID-19 cases and deaths even with lockdowns.[2] But the predicted surge didn't come[3]—thank God. Unfortunately, we had devastated our economy and harmed millions because we trusted the predictions.

President Trump had prepared the nation for war-scale casualties. Military personnel were sent out to each state to help. "They're going to war," he said. "Nobody has seen this [many casualties] since 1917, which was the greatest of them all...up to a hundred million people killed."[4]

We waited. But the promised apocalypse never happened. Hospitals across the country that were supposed to be filled—if not overflowing—with the critically ill were mostly empty. Even in New York, which experts predicted would need 140,000 hospital beds, only about 18,500 were in use.[5] Many thousands of field-hospital beds that had been brought in by ship or laid out in temporary shelters sat empty. The USNS *Comfort*, which had docked in Manhattan in late March to help with the overflow, departed at the end of April, unneeded.[6] One field hospital in Brooklyn, the *New York Post* noted, cost $21 million to build and "never saw a patient."[7]

This is what prompted the big pivot. Within a few weeks the mantra changed from "flatten the curve" to "stop the spread." Just a short time before, no one had thought we could stop the spread, as a Live Science article from March 16 explained: "Health officials take for granted that COVID-19 will continue to infect millions of people around the world over the coming weeks and months.... A flatter curve...assumes the same number of people ultimately get infected, but over a longer period of time."[8]

So, expert opinion contradicted "stop the spread," but now that we've done the experiment, what does the evidence say? Is there any clear evidence that our drastic measures slowed or stopped the spread of the coronavirus?

If lockdowns could really alter the course of this pandemic, then coronavirus case counts should have shown a big drop whenever and wherever lockdowns took place. The effect should have been obvious, though with a time lag. It takes time for new coronavirus infections to be officially counted, so we would expect the numbers to plummet as soon as the waiting time was over. How long? New infections should plummet on day one and be noticed about ten or eleven days from the lockdown. By day six, the number of people with first symptoms of infection should plummet (six days is the average time for symptoms to appear).[9] By day nine or ten, far fewer people would be heading to doctors with worsening symptoms. If COVID-19 tests were performed right away, we would expect the positives to drop dramatically on day ten or eleven (assuming quick turnarounds on tests). That's when the lights would go out on the coronavirus.

Is that what we saw? The United Kingdom is a good test case. On March 23, Prime Minister Boris Johnson made a sudden course change and announced a police-enforced lockdown in response to COVID-19.[10]

Before that, the UK had been taking a relaxed approach—like Sweden. If ever there was a flipped policy switch, this was it. So did the lights go out on coronavirus in the UK, or at least dramatically dim?

Not at all. Figure 9.1 shows the daily confirmed coronavirus cases in the UK from the start of March through mid-May. We're using a logarithmic plot here to make it easier to see the exponential growth we talked about in chapter 8. We want to focus not on the numbers but on the shape of the curve. Specifically, the changing *slope* of the curve indicates the changing value of R_e.

We haven't smoothed the data because we want to stick with reported numbers. That means we have to look at the overall path without being distracted by all the jags. When we do that (with the help of the dotted lines) we see a steep upward slope through mid-March, which indicates a value of R_e well above one. But notice that the slope already appears to

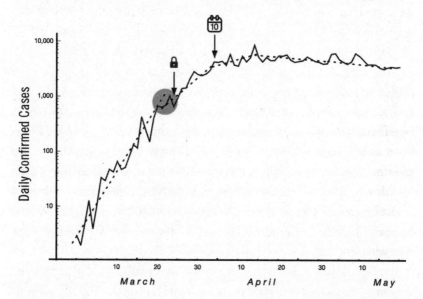

Figure 9.1. Daily confirmed COVID-19 cases in the UK. The lock marks the date of the lockdown. The day-10 calendar shows where cases should have plummeted if the lockdown stopped the spread. Dashed line segments (placed by hand) are a visual aid for seeing the change of slope. The grey circle marks the first visual downward change of slope. Data from https://ourworldindata.org.[11]

be decreasing—which means R_e was dropping—before the lockdown went into effect. Although the number of new cases per day continued to grow until it peaked in mid-April, R_e was steadily falling the whole time. This means the spread of the virus was visibly inhibited by around March 20—several days before Johnson ordered the lockdown and two weeks before that order could have had a visible effect.

The stark change on March 23 in how Britons lived caused no stark change in the curve. No sudden step-like drop in new cases. No sign of a flipped switch. Instead, we see more of the slow-and-steady downward trend in the slope that had started before the lockdown.

Of course, we can imagine that the curve could have looked worse without the lockdown. But this is storytelling. The actual numbers show no clear break in the trend where it clearly should have broken if the lockdown had altered the course of the outbreak. If the line had leveled off around the ten-day marker, that would be a break in the trend. Likewise, if the curve bent sharply downward near that point, that would also break the trend. Instead, it chugs along as though nothing changed.

Figure 9.2 shows what we mean by breaks in the trend. Here we compare the cumulative daily counts of coronavirus cases in the UK and China. Again, the ten-day marker shows where we should see any effects of the UK lockdown. The plateaus in the grey curve are clear breaks in the trend—points where the reported daily cases in China plunged and remained low for some time. This is likely due to unreliable reporting. Whatever the cause, we can see abrupt changes in the numerical trend in the data from China. If lockdowns could also cause abrupt changes, we should see one around April 2 (where the ten-day marker is) in the data from the UK. But we don't.

A UK policy other than the lockdown probably did affect the numbers, but not abruptly. At the start of April, the British government announced the goal of processing one hundred thousand COVID-19 tests per day by the end of the month, a ten-fold expansion.[12] As a result, the number of tests performed each day vastly exceeded the number of people with new symptoms. This changed the effective meaning of "new cases." At first, it meant sick people who were tested and found to have the virus. By May it mostly meant people with mild or no symptoms who were being tested *en masse* as a way of tracking the pandemic. The far right end of the curve in Figure 9.1 is probably artificially high as a result, though we don't think this affects our conclusions.

There's one more thing that's clear from the UK numbers. As of mid-May, the coronavirus had infected over *two hundred thousand* people in the UK since the lockdown went into effect (taking the lag into account). And that's just the recorded cases. Since about 80 percent of infections cause mild or no symptoms,[13] the vast majority of infected people likely went untested and therefore unrecorded. This means the real number of infections in the UK after lockdown can easily have been over a million.

So the lockdown didn't come close to stopping the spread.

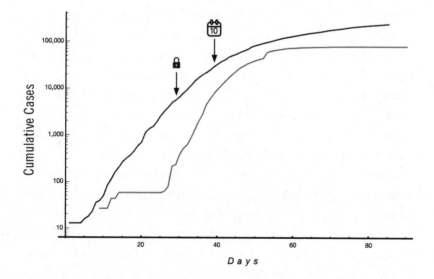

Figure 9.2. Cumulative daily cases in the UK (black line) and China (grey line) over a period of about 80 days. Start and end dates differ for the two countries. (The point of the figure is to compare the visual shapes.)

COMPARING STATES

Although President Trump's critics accuse him of wanting to consolidate power, he respected the federal structure of our political system during the pandemic. This meant that states handled the lockdown, with some counties and cities also playing a role. Supreme Court justice Louis Brandeis famously called the states "laboratories of democracy." Different states can test out different policies, and they can learn from each other. That proved true in 2020; we can now compare the outcome in different states, each of which had its own approach.

And what do we find? As in the UK, mandated lockdowns seem to have had little effect on the spread of the coronavirus. Though no state did a 180-degree policy change like the one in the UK, the curves are broadly similar. Figure 9.3 shows the daily case curves for the United States as a whole and for thirteen U.S. states. As for the UK, we consistently see a steep climb as the virus spreads unhindered, followed by a transition (marked by the grey circles) to a flatter curve. At some point, the curves always slope downward, though this isn't obvious for all states as of May 20.

Again, the lockdowns can't be the cause of these transitions. In the first place, the transition happened even in places without lockdown orders (see Iowa and Arkansas). And where there were lockdowns, the transitions tended to occur well before the lockdowns could have had any effect (just as we saw for the UK). The only possible exceptions are California, which on March 19 became the first state to be locked down,[14] and Connecticut, which followed four days later.

Even in these places, though, the downward transitions probably started before the lockdowns could have altered the curves. The reason is that our assumed one-day turnaround for COVID-19 test results probably wasn't met in either state. On March 30, the *Los Angeles Times* reported the turnaround time to be eight days.[15] That would make the delay from infection to confirmation not the ten we assumed but more like seventeen days (six for symptoms to appear, three for them to develop, eight for test processing). In early April, the *Hartford Courant* reported similar problems with delayed test results in Connecticut.[16]

And once more, there's no decisive drop on the dates when lockdowns should have changed the course of the curves. Instead the curves gradually bend downward for reasons that pre-date the lockdowns, with no clear changes ten days later. Anyone who wants to think the lockdowns worked could say that the curves would have been higher after the ten-day points without them, but that's wishful thinking. We can't redo history to prove them wrong. The point is that the sudden and dramatic changes we should see if they were right aren't there. If we showed lockdown fans these curves without any markings, they wouldn't be able to tell when or even if the lockdowns went into effect.

The vertical lines mark the date when the number of deaths attributed to the coronavirus reached five per million people in the population. This is probably the best way to mark similar extents of viral progress in each state, since we don't know how many total cases there were. The curves usually start to bend somewhere around the same death toll (roughly five per million people), which suggests that the approach of herd immunity caused the bends. In other words, we see in Figure 9.3 not only a lack of evidence that lockdowns caused the curves to bend but also evidence of the true cause: the very early stages of herd immunity.

In fact, a May 18 column in the *New York Times*[17] argued that coronavirus cases in New York City probably peaked before the state lockdown began on March 22. Though that newspaper is not known for taking a critical stance on lockdowns, this point implies that the spread was slowing before the mayor and governor even ordered the lockdown.

We can see this better by going back to the death curves of Figure 6.5. Deaths attributed to the coronavirus across all age groups clearly peaked in mid-April before falling. We presume that the (much higher) true infection curves would be of similar shape, though peaking earlier. All the problems we've discussed about testing make the new-case curves in Figure 9.3 less reliable than the death curves in Figure 6.5. Taken together, though, they give a consistent picture.

Something caused this overall decline in deaths, and it can't have been lockdowns, which weren't maintained (or heeded) in full force through June. At the moment, we can only speculate. But if this virus is like others, the causes of the decline are likely some mix of changing seasons and the gradual onset of herd immunity.

The panic and sweeping lockdowns, which did little, were a big mistake.

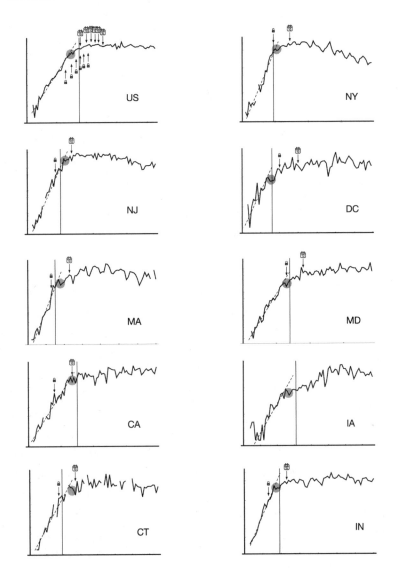

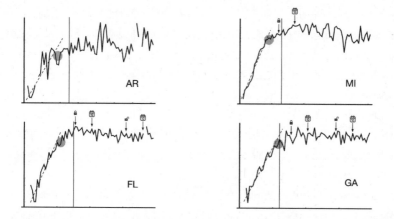

Figure 9.3. Daily confirmed COVID-19 cases for the whole United States and thirteen individual states (logarithmic plots) up to May 20, 2020. Dashed line segments (placed by hand) show the initial steep increase with grey circles marking the first visual downward change of slope. As in Figure 9.1, locks mark the lockdown dates, and ten-day calendars show where lockdowns would have had visible effects. Open locks mark when lockdowns ended for Florida and Georgia, both in the first wave of states to emerge from lockdown. The vertical lines mark the dates when deaths attributed to the coronavirus reached five per million people in the population. Gaps in curves are the result of unreported data. Information sources: https://ourworldindata.org (for U.S. cases); https://covidtracking.com/api (for state cases); https://www.nytimes.com/interactive/2020/us/coronavirus-stay-at-home-order.html (for lockdown dates).[18]

WORLD TOUR

We can also examine the effects of lockdowns by looking at different countries.

The United States contains about four percent of the world population. Yet from late April through mid-May, our country claimed to have about a third of the reported coronavirus cases and a quarter to a third of related deaths worldwide. What accounts for these mismatches?

The Philippines, with 107 million people, has a population about a third the size of the U.S. On May 12, 2020, they reported 11,086 cases and 726 deaths, according to Worldometer.[19] This amounts to 104 cases and 7 deaths per million people. On that same day, the

United States reported 4,187 cases and 247 deaths per million—40 and 35 times higher than the Philippines! Lockdowns in the two countries were broadly similar. Both had various and sundry restrictions, with Manila reportedly facing the strictest measures, like some areas in the U.S.[20]

One clear difference was the rate of COVID-19 testing, which was much higher in the United States. According to Worldometer, the United States carried out twenty-nine thousand tests per million; the Philippines, only sixteen hundred per million.[21]

Perhaps the United States was quicker to ascribe deaths to the coronavirus. Weather may also have mattered. The Philippines enjoys warmer and sunnier weather than the U.S. danger zones—the New York, Chicago, and Detroit metro areas. A late spring, with cool temperatures and heavy rain, hit much of the United States.

On that same date, May 12, Taiwan, a country of 24 million people, had 440 cases and 7 deaths. That works out to a mere 0.3 deaths per million, with *no lockdowns*. Sweden was discussed frequently in the news because of their modest measures. They had 2,641 reported cases and 322 deaths per million, a far higher rate than Taiwan's. Again, weather could have been a factor—helpful in Taiwan and not so helpful in Sweden.

Belgium has about as many people as Sweden, 11.5 million, though more spread out. They had 53,449 reported cases and 8,707 reported deaths, or 4,612 and 751 per million respectively. Those are the worst per-capita numbers of all countries for May 12 (and for many dates before and after)—three times the U.S. figures. The Belgian lockdown measures were a lot like the American ones, though probably more strictly enforced because of the country's smaller size.[22]

If we categorize countries by their per-capita coronavirus deaths on May 12 and focus on countries with at least a million people, twelve reported more than one hundred deaths per million. In this unenviable category were, from worst to best: Belgium, Spain, Italy, UK, France,

Sweden, Netherlands, Ireland, the United States, Switzerland, Canada, and Portugal. All but Sweden had lockdowns of varying severity, and even Sweden imposed modest restrictions.

In the next best category, with reported death rates from eleven to ninety-nine per million, were thirty-one countries. These included, from worst to best: Denmark (ninety-two deaths per million), Germany (ninety-one), Iran (eighty), Norway (forty-one), Israel (thirty), Mexico (twenty-eight), Russia (fourteen), and Greece (fourteen). Lockdowns in those countries varied widely, as we'll see.

Better still, with reported death rates from one to ten per million, were fifty-one countries. These included Japan (with modest measures but no lockdown), South Korea (with more stringent measures and also no lockdown), both at five per million, Singapore, Malaysia, Afghanistan, Georgia, Jamaica, Costa Rica, Paraguay, India, China, and a host of African countries.

Finally, in the top category, thirty countries reported deaths under one per million. These included Thailand, Taiwan, Jordan, Hong Kong, Botswana, Syria, Myanmar, Ethiopia, and so on.[23]

Enough of the numbers. Let's do the comparison with pictures. To do this, we checked each country to see which had a government-imposed lockdown of at least half their population at any time in late winter or early spring 2020.[24] Oxford University compiled a coronavirus "government response tracker" which tracked dates of lockdowns and tried to quantify the "stringency" of responses.[25] This database has more detail than ours, but differs little on the substance of whether lockdowns were used. Their database also investigates about forty fewer countries than ours. Comparing our data to theirs changes none of our conclusions.

Governments embraced lockdowns with gusto the world over. On April 3, 2020, not long after the start of the crisis, Euro News was able to report, "Half of Humanity Now on Lockdown as 90 Countries Call for Confinement."[26] Half of humanity—"more than 3.9 billion people"! If lockdowns were the right call, then this is impressive.

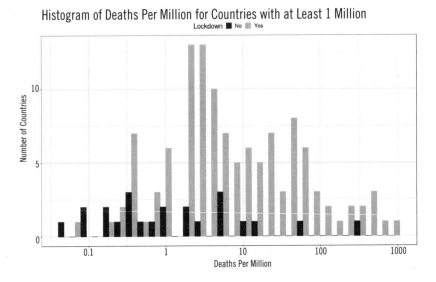

Figure 9.4. A count of countries with various total reported coronavirus deaths per million as of May 12, 2020 (for countries with at least a million people).

Figure 9.4 shows a histogram of the deaths per million for those countries with a population of at least one million, distinguishing countries with lockdowns from those without. The death rates across the different countries are on the horizontal axis. These ranged from zero (for Vietnam) to almost one thousand per million. The bar heights show how many countries had the specified death rate.

The horizontal scale is by log base ten, a necessity because of the huge variability in death rates. Countries that did not have lockdowns are in black; those with lockdowns are grey. If anything, the countries without lockdowns tend to be further to the left. That is, they had lower death rates.

Now, there are so many factors at play here, and not that many countries without lockdowns. So, this evidence doesn't prove that lockdowns didn't work. Rather, it shows how hard it is to show that they did work. And that's a serious problem when we consider the full costs of shutting economies down. We'll unpack those costs in chapter 10, but as a quick spoiler: they're *brutally high*.

Another way to look at it, since population density may play a role, is a plot of the death rate per million by population size. Again, we limit our graph to countries with at least one million people.

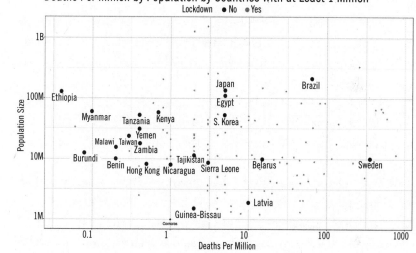

Figure 9.5. Coronavirus deaths per million (long axis) arranged by population (short axis) as of May 12, 2020 (for countries with at least a million people).

Again, countries that remained open are in black, and those that shut down are in grey. The two top population points are, of course, China and India. The countries with the highest death rates were discussed above. Death rates were more than highly variable: they were all over the place![27]

Lockdowns ranged from severe, as in China's Wuhan, to practically non-existent or highly localized, as in Botswana, where major cities saw greater control than the countryside and smaller cities.[28]

If lockdowns had determined the course of the coronavirus, then we would not expect to see such vast variability in the reported death rates across the world. Belgium had 751 deaths per million while Ethiopia, population 109.2 million, had the lowest reported non-zero death rate of 0.04 per million. This is a 19-thousand-fold difference.

Ethiopia did declare a state of emergency, but it had no lockdown.[29] The United States sent the country a "$37m package which encompassed case management, infection prevention and control, laboratory strengthening, public health screening, and communications and media campaigns, among others."[30]

Vietnam, population 95.5 million, acted early to quarantine people exposed and infected, but did not have a national lockdown. A reported 18,000 businesses were forced to close, but the country had zero reported deaths.[31]

Sweden, which had no lockdown, did better than the UK and six other countries that did have lockdowns. South Dakota, which had no lockdown, did seven times better than Chicago (or all of Illinois), which did.

Brazil did not have a countrywide lockdown, but a handful of cities threatened to seize control, and some did carry out local measures. The same kind of thing happened in the United States, with harsh mandatory measures in what the mainstream press portrayed as more enlightened cities, to nothing in some flyover states. Japan had no lockdown and did fine, relatively speaking. The press ignores the Land of the Rising Sun, though. Wonder why? In Georgia (the country), only Tbilisi seems to have been locked down.

Some countries locked down only a few major cities or ports, others cut off foreign travel and either left their citizens alone or only issued warnings. Some lockdowns were especially harsh, with food shortages happening fast, as in Paraguay. Lithuania required people to wear coronavirus bracelets to indicate their health status. Foreign workers in Qatar were made to huddle in lockdowns in camps. Albania used drones to find lockdown scofflaws. Even nomads in Western Sahara were ordered to stay in their tents.

There seems to be a trend toward lower death rates in hotter countries, and in the warmer areas of large countries such as the United States.

Population density also likely played a role. It's easier for a virus to spread in tightly packed quarters. Australia and New Zealand both locked down, and both had four-per-million death rates, but then it was summer in both places at the start of the pandemic. They also hadn't begun their usual flu season (and neither had other Southern Hemisphere countries).

We can't dismiss population density either. England's Office of National Statistics issued a study that showed a strong correlation between the death rate and overcrowding in housing units. The death rate was (relatively) small when the overcrowding was slight, and large when it was extreme. The enforced stay-at-home orders, quarantining the healthy and sick together, may have encouraged the spread of the disease.[32]

Countries differ as much as people do: average age and health of citizens. Masks worn or not. Different health-care resources of every kind. Different levels of compliance with mitigation. In some countries there was not as much oversight on lockdowns, and even in those without lockdowns authorities took some measures, as in Taiwan. In Guinea, police fired on lockdown protesters. In Somalia police fired and hit their targets, killing protesters.

Reporting also varied wildly. The West went with earnest, hour-by-hour updates for every number. We hardly heard from, or about, African countries. And most were skeptical of reporting from totalitarian states such as Iran and North Korea.

Tajikistan only reported a few deaths (two per million), which some said was a lie. Maybe. Who knows? Everybody is sure China lied. Did Japan? Did Belarus? They didn't lock down. Meanwhile, over-counting and excessive fear blurred the numbers in the West.

So, what can we conclude from this survey of countries? Only one thing: we do not know that lockdowns worked, that is, that they reduced deaths. We can't prove the opposite either—that they made no difference in the death rate. But the proof has to rest with those who would call for lockdowns. Otherwise, almost any claim of a looming disaster becomes a ready excuse to proclaim something like martial law, provided a few experts can be lined up to warn that the sky is falling. To justify their calls for lockdowns, advocates need to show—not just assume—that lockdowns really do save enough lives to justify the human cost. They haven't done that.

On the contrary: several no-lockdown countries had low death rates. Given the low death rates in several of the no-lockdown countries and states, and the graphs showing the death rate curves and the lack of any meaningful correlation between lockdown orders and case curves, it will be almost impossible to prove that the lockdowns made much difference.[33]

THE BOTTOM LINE

As we'll see in the next chapter, shutting down the economy had huge costs—in both money and lives. So we'd like to think it was worth it. But if the economic and human costs vastly outstripped the benefits, we need to face that fact and chart a better course, should something like this pandemic happen again, as it surely will.[34]

As much as we would like to think we saved millions of lives by "stopping the spread," the facts say otherwise. As we mentioned in chapter 8, months before the politics of COVID-19 kicked in, WHO weighed the merits of social distancing and lockdowns and found them wanting.[35] On top of that, as we've seen in this chapter, daily new case counts show the spread was already slowing before the shutdowns, both in the UK (Figure 9.1) and in the U.S. (Figure 9.3). Respiratory viruses for which we have no vaccines (including most causes of common colds) tend to quell themselves by spreading.[36] Never before had lockdowns of such a scale been tried. Why, then, did we think we could halt the coronavirus this way?

In any case, we've now run the experiment. We were the guinea pigs. And there's no evidence that the coronavirus paid any attention to our efforts.

New York governor Andrew Cuomo started grappling with this painful truth in early May, when he realized that thousands of housebound New

Yorkers were catching the bug. CNBC News noted that these findings seemed "to clash with Cuomo's prior assurances that isolation can reliably prevent transmission."[37] Yes, they did. Back in April Cuomo had said, "I was afraid that it was going to infect my family no matter what I did. We're past that.... If you isolate, if you take the precautions, your family won't get infected."[38] By "past that," he meant that he had moved past the "flatten the curve" mantra and on to the "stop the spread" mantra.

By May, he had moved past both.

"Much of this comes down to what you do to protect yourself," Cuomo said on May 6. "Everything is closed down, government has done everything it could, society has done everything it could. Now it's up to you."[39] Hmm. So, in a land where government is supposed to be of the people, for the people, and by the people, centralized power was exercised in a way that caused great harm to the people, in the name of saving lives. And when it became evident that it had all been for naught, the new advice was, "Take care of yourself."

Really?

How are we to make sense of all this? What we said at the start of chapter 8 is surely true. Viruses spread by physical transfer from the infected to the susceptible. So in theory we could stop them from spreading by staying apart and taking other extreme precautions. In practice, though, we live together in societies that will never be sterile. Respiratory viruses are a part of life, and that's not going to change.

Maybe it's hard for us to flatten the curve or hinder the spread of the virus with extreme social distancing and lockdowns because we already achieve most of the benefits from the moderate precautions that we have always taken. We always take commonsense precautions to avoid catching and spreading bugs. We react to news in ways that fit the details of our individual lives. The curve only gets so flat, though, before we reach a point of diminishing returns. Every now and then technology delivers a game changer—the germ theory of disease, vaccines, antibiotics, X-rays. A real quarantine—isolating carriers of deadly communicable diseases—has been a game changer, but universal lockdown never was.

It comes down to rapidly escalating costs for rapidly diminishing returns. We don't want to become misanthropic hermits in hazmat suits. There's far more to life than safety, real or illusory. And, as we'll see in the next chapter, when we forget that we may do far more harm than good.

CHAPTER 10

THE HUMAN COST

*The cost of a thing is the amount of what I will call life
which is required to be exchanged for it, immediately or
in the long run.*

—*Henry David Thoreau*[1]

Everything we do has a cost. That's life in a world of scarcity—of health care, time, money, and any other finite resource. We can't avoid such scarcity even in a world of ever more abundance. That's why our choices involve trade-offs. Those trade-offs don't disappear because lives are at risk. That just raises the stakes.

We have seen what the benefits of our panic-induced coronavirus response were supposed to be. And we've seen that they weren't anything like what they were supposed to be.

Now we want to know: What were the *costs* of our response? The total costs, of course, go beyond dollars. They include lives, life-years, suffering, loss of freedom, and so on. We can be no more precise than the subject matter allows. In some cases, we'll need to settle for a simple list of costs, without pretending to attach numbers. Still, wherever possible, we would like rough estimates.

Let's start with dollars and move from there to the flesh-and-blood impact on human lives.

In Dollars

To figure out the net financial cost of the measures we took against the coronavirus, we need some sense of what a more normal response would have cost U.S. taxpayers, without the panic and forced shutdown. After all, the coronavirus didn't shut down businesses. Governments did.

Imagine that state and national governments around the world had carried on business as usual. We don't mean they did nothing. They just did what they usually do for epidemics and pandemics. Imagine that agencies like WHO and the CDC had treated the coronavirus as they would treat a really bad strain of the flu—reporting what they knew and admitting what they didn't know. And imagine the media had seen their job as simply reporting the facts, calmly and fairly. (Yes, imagining that will take some doing.) In that scenario, there would have been far less cause for the public to panic and for politicians to overreact.

Obviously, the pandemic itself would have cost us a lot, in terms of death, sickness, losses in productivity, financial and psychological wellbeing, and so forth. But, as we argued in the previous two chapters, there is no clear evidence the panic and shutdowns actually reduced that cost.

So what we want to know is how much our unprecedented response cost us, *over and above* the costs we would have borne anyway. Only by subtracting what the pandemic would have cost in any case can we get a fair estimate of the cost of our response.

But how do we figure out what the pandemic would have cost without the extreme response? By "extreme response," we don't mean the normal stuff we would have done voluntarily if there had been no panic—social distancing, wearing good masks when at high risk of infection, working from home where possible, extra hand washing, and the like—which we assume confers some benefit. We mean the widespread panic, costly shelter-in-place orders, blanket quarantines, closing businesses, closing churches, snitching on neighbors, arresting dads who played with their kids in the park, and so forth. We do none of these things in response to the flu, even in a bad flu season. We've never done them even during a flu pandemic. So, the baseline cost would be costs of the virus itself plus a non-panicked response.

One way to estimate this is to look at the cost of the flu in an average season. Depending upon how we count it, the flu costs the United States between ten and one hundred billion dollars per year.[2] Let's take the mean and go with fifty-five billion dollars. Understand that this is a highly uncertain number. We're just trying to get in the ballpark.

Next, let's assume that no one who died from COVID-19 would have gotten sick or died from any other cause in 2020. In reality, the people most vulnerable to death from the coronavirus were also disproportionately vulnerable to death from other causes—old people already in ill health. Thus, some who died from the coronavirus almost surely would have died from other causes if there had been no coronavirus. But to avoid any risk that we undercount the costs of the coronavirus itself (and thus exaggerate the cost of the extreme response to it), we'll ignore that.

For the same reason, let's assume that the coronavirus was fully four times worse than the flu, and thus justified a more costly response. (In terms of deaths, it was likely closer to half again as bad as the 2018 flu season, though distributed more heavily to the old and infirm.) That would be a $220 billion punch to the U.S. economy. Even in an age where "trillion" rolls loosely off the tongue, $220 billion is a lot of money—roughly five times the 2018 budget of the Department of Homeland Security.

Still, the U.S. economy is roughly a hundred times that size and was humming along well up through February 2020. As a result, we doubt this extra hit would have caused a recession, though it would have swelled the federal deficit some and might have slowed economic growth.

Now, one could argue that the cost doesn't scale that simply: four times more deaths and illnesses could have far more than four times the impact on the economy. Maybe. But that four times figure is very generous. Besides, for all we know, the marginal economic costs might diminish. That is, the first fifty thousand cases of the disease might cost more financially than the next fifty thousand. As we've seen, despite the dire warnings, we didn't swamp our healthcare system nationwide. Quite the opposite: the coronavirus response has created economic depression in the health-care sector, as we diverted resources to the pandemic and suspended "elective" medical procedures. So, since we've already been very liberal in assigning costs, we don't see any good reason not to stick with the $220 billion estimate.

Another way to derive this figure would be to use the economic measure of a life-year. Contrary to what you may think, economists don't simply decide among themselves what the years of our lives are worth. They assume (plausibly) that losing, say, ten years of your life is worse than losing one year. And then they look at how much society is willing to spend to save years of life by reducing risk. They look at things like the cost of smoke detectors, airbags, and helmets; the premium for working dangerous jobs; and the like. We're not calculating the value of a person's life, but rather how much we value reducing the risk of losing our lives or the lives of loved ones.

Estimates vary, of course. But at the moment, a life year seems to run about $150,000 in the United States. Don't sweat the details for now. We'll come back to this issue later. Here we just want an estimate of the cost of the coronavirus pandemic minus the shutdowns. "Applying that measure [$150,000 per life year] to the age distribution of the deceased," notes health policy expert Geoffrey Joyce, "and adding the costs of treating the infected population, the total cost of COVID-19 in the U.S. under current restrictions appears to be about $150 billion."[3] He wrote that at the end of April. If we add the deaths from May and June to the total, we end up with a number very close to our first estimate: $220 billion, give or take.

A third and final way to rough out what the pandemic would have cost if we had met it with a normal, voluntary response would be to compare it to the economic cost of the 1918 Spanish flu pandemic, which killed (roughly) 675,000 Americans. There were social distancing policies in 1918, but nothing as extreme as in 2020. So, with the proper adjustments for population and inflation, we could estimate the cost of the 2020 pandemic if we had stuck with equally modest policies.

A number of studies have tried to nail down the cost of the Spanish flu pandemic, which killed far more people than the coronavirus.[4] It seems to have packed an economic punch in the short run, but recovery came quickly. A survey of the literature by the St. Louis Fed put it this way: "Most of the evidence indicates that the economic effects of the 1918 influenza pandemic were short-term."[5] Alas, solid numbers are hard to come by.

One April 2020 study, though, analyzed the 1918 pandemic for the purpose of applying its lessons to current events.[6] Its three authors, two at the Fed and one at MIT, argued that it was the 1918 pandemic itself, and not the "public health interventions," that depressed the economy. They also said that "cities that intervened earlier and more aggressively do not perform worse and, if anything, grow faster after the pandemic is over." The interventions included social distancing and limits on large crowds.

Again, it's hard to draw strong conclusions from the patchy historical records, but the press loved the implications.[7] If nothing else, they offered a handy cudgel for whacking Donald Trump, who was concerned at the time that the "cure" not be worse than the disease.

But how is this relevant to the 2020 pandemic? The 1918 responses were more akin to the moderate Swedish response in 2020. Efforts were local and organic, not national and imposed from above. Woodrow Wilson, the president at the time, seems to have paid the pandemic no mind; historians "have been unable to find a single occasion on which he mentioned [the Spanish flu] in public."[8] So, the study did nothing to show that the extreme response mandated by national, state, and local governments that we saw *in 2020* will be better for local economies than more modest alternatives, however much its authors wanted readers to draw that conclusion.

So let's return now to our $220 billion figure as our generous estimate for the cost of the pandemic if there had been no lockdown. What did the lockdown cost us above that? Economists will be busy answering this question for a long time, since there are all sorts of knock-on costs that will reverberate for years. Still, we can point to one big bill that was entered on the federal ledger right away. The so-called "stimulus" bill signed by the president on March 27 was about $2.2 trillion. One could argue that, with extra tax relief, it amounted to $800 billion dollars more than that.[9] But to avoid inflating the costs, let's ignore that, treating it instead as a transfer payment from the future to the present. That would mean that the response cost us almost two trillion dollars right off the bat (subtracting, as we said above, the $220 billion.)

Remember, this is money borrowed to try to fill the hole we dug in the economy by our response to the coronavirus. It represents goods and services, with accompanying wages and salaries, that we couldn't produce because of the lockdown.

That $2 trillion, though, is probably the minimum financial cost for a lockdown that lasts a couple of months. Credit Suisse projected that the U.S. economy would lose (if annualized) a third of its value in the second quarter of 2020.[10] Another analysis estimated the cost of the shutdown to be about 5 percent of the GDP per month.[11] All three figures point to a lockdown cost of about a trillion dollars per month. Even in July, the bitter ends of the lockdowns lingered. The minimum cost to the U.S. economy from the lockdown, then, is at least several trillion dollars.[12] For comparison, the budget for the federal government for all of 2019 was $4.4 trillion—larger than any other government in the world. If we limit the cost of our response to the coronavirus to, say, six months in 2020, that means it may be the steepest bill we will ever pay.

MASSIVE UNEMPLOYMENT

Adding up dollars like this can make it look as if we're treating money as the only thing that matters. But that's an illusion. We care about dollars not because dollars matter in themselves, but because they serve as a means and a measure of a host of human goods. Lost dollars mean lost businesses, lost jobs, lost innovations that enhance and extend lives, lost years, even lost lives. The dollars are really a proxy for these more important things. But we can also forget the dollars and talk about the things that really matter to us.

Like jobs. Even analysts who think the debate is between dollars on one side and lives on the other know that the shutdown devastated the economy and cost tens of millions of jobs. We mentioned the dismal numbers in the introduction. In February, unemployment in the United States was at a historic low of 3.5 percent. The week ending March 28 saw 6.9 million new jobless claims. The next week added 5.2 million jobless claims. The next week, 6.6 million new jobless claims, then another 4.4 million.[13] And for the week ending May 2, another 3.2 million. That's 33.5 million new jobless claims over a mere seven-week period. There has never been anything like this in American history. Ever. By the end of May, the new jobless claims had climbed to nearly 41 million.[14] Remember, many of the people who lost their jobs have spouses and children that depend on them. It's no surprise that hunger and food insecurity surged within weeks.

This tsunami of joblessness did not wash evenly over the country. If you were already embedded in the digital economy, or you could do your job online in a pinch, you may have stayed dry during the first wave. If you worked in leisure or hospitality—for a hotel, airline, restaurant, conference service, or in entertainment—you were the first to find yourself underwater.

Remember the worry about COVID-19 overwhelming our health-care system? That didn't happen. Instead, the sector saw massive job losses. By early May, over 1.4 million jobs were lost in health care.[15]

Jobs in retail and manufacturing were also hit hard—though warehouse clubs and supercenters actually added jobs because the powers that be declared them essential.[16] Small family-owned businesses without much margin closed. It's anyone's guess how many will return.

To make a long story short, the lockdown hit the people and businesses that could least afford it the hardest. Some of this might have happened with no lockdown. Even Sweden has suffered a (much smaller) slowdown, since it's part of the global economy.[17] Still, we can safely say that forty million Americans lost their jobs because of the lockdown. If you don't like thinking in terms of trillions of dollars, then think instead about forty million income earners becoming unemployed, many with dependents, and many already low-income earners.

DEATHS OF DESPAIR

Dan Bongino is a former Secret Service agent turned commentator. On April 21, he tweeted that a close friend had killed himself after being "let go" from his job because of the shutdown.[18] That's one person. But how many times did we hear individual stories reported in a way that made the case for stricter measures, without hearing about those who would suffer under them?

One physician, Nicole Saphier, saw Bongino's heartfelt lament and made some back-of-the-envelope calculations.[19] "As unemployment approaches 20%," she tweeted, "each 1% rise can result in 3.3% spike in drug OD [overdoses]/ 1% increase in suicides (National Bureau of Economic Research). If unemployment hits 32%, ~77,000 Americans may die as a result. Will economic fallout mortality be greater than the virus itself?"

ABC News reported from the San Francisco Bay area, "Doctors at John Muir Medical Center in Walnut Creek say they have seen more deaths by suicide during this quarantine period than deaths from the COVID-19 virus."[20] One doctor said he'd "seen a year's worth of suicide attempts in the last four weeks."

The New York Post reported on coronavirus-related suicides.[21] Other outlets reported a surge in deaths from opioids and alcohol, which are often tied to joblessness.[22]

We have collected dozens of such stories from around the United States, Europe, India, and New Zealand. These are anecdotes, but scientific studies suggest that they are harbingers of what's to come.

In early April, the *Journal of the American Medical Association* (JAMA) was already warning that "the potential for adverse outcomes on suicide risk is high." They based that judgment on past "economic downturns," which "are usually associated with higher suicide rates compared with periods of relative prosperity."[23] Enforced isolation and closed religious services, they argued, would also increase suicidal thoughts and suicides.

A meta-analysis (an analysis of multiple published studies) in the *World Journal of Psychiatry* confirmed that finding.[24] "Economic recession periods," it concluded, "appear to increase overall suicide rates."

Another contemporary report asked, "How does the coronavirus pandemic affect suicide rates?"[25] The authors noted, "Although data on numbers of calls specifically related to COVID-19 distress are not yet available for the National Suicide Prevention Lifeline, during March 2020, the Disaster Distress Helpline saw a 338 percent increase in call volume compared with February 2020." Callers reported feelings of isolation and severe anxiety. The *Daily Mail* noted that the Los Angeles suicide prevention hotline received seventy-five times more calls in March than in the previous month.[26]

Confirming Saphier's tweet in April, a study published in May estimated that the shutdowns could ultimately lead to seventy-five thousand such deaths.[27] Another detailed analysis suggested that anxiety alone could cost seven times more life-years than could be saved by the lockdowns.[28]

We can't yet prove that pandemic panic led to net spikes in these deaths of despair. Still, the stories started appearing at once, even in media outlets that supported the lockdowns. And based on what we know of past economic disasters, we have no doubt what the evidence will show.

The exact toll could be immense. Many suicides could come far after the crisis has subsided, since the effects of the lockdowns will linger for years. Deaths from the coronavirus are being noted and seen. The deaths of despair caused by our response will scatter across the years, mostly unseen.

DEATHS FROM EXTREME POVERTY

In every country, no matter how prosperous, some people are on the edge. Imagine we ranked every American adult by income. There would be people in the bottom 10 percent, the bottom 5 percent, and the bottom one percent. Any change for the worse—a tsunami, an earthquake, a pandemic, a depression—would hurt these people the most. They don't have any margin. They can't just pivot, or move, or draw down their savings, or cash out a 401k, or sell the boat.

Now consider a country much poorer than the United States, one where millions of people still live on a couple of dollars a day. What do you think a global depression will do to them?

On May 11, the *L.A. Times* said outright what we had been thinking for over two months: "The economic devastation the pandemic wreaks on the ultra-poor could ultimately kill more people than the virus itself." Of course, the story blamed the pandemic itself. And it should get some of the blame. But the panic that followed in its wake should get the lion's share.

That fact is clear from the story. It was not about millions of poor people dying from COVID-19. It was about millions of poor people dying from the response to COVID-19. "Hunger," the story noted, "is already rising in the poorest parts of the world, where lockdowns and social distancing measures have erased incomes and put even basic food items out of reach."

This is even more depressing because of the progress made over the past three decades in ridding the world of such desperate poverty. "Since 1990," the *LA Times* story observed, "more than 1 billion people—13% of the world's population—have risen out of extreme poverty, according to the World Bank."

At the beginning of 2020, 734 million people were in extreme poverty. The UN now predicts that the events of 2020 could "plunge as many as 420 million [more] people into extreme poverty, defined as earning less than $2 a day." David Beasley, executive director of the United Nations World Food Programme, predicted that shocks to food supply chains could lead to 300,000 deaths per day.[29] In other words, more people around the world could die every two days from our response to the pandemic than those who died from the entire pandemic itself.

There's no way to nail down exact numbers, but the ones cited above are surely in the ballpark. And since the lockdowns happened almost everywhere, the well-off people who give to poverty-fighting religious ministries and relief organizations will be hard-pressed to help.

What about the poor in the United States? We have a safety net, and surplus wealth. For the most part even our poor do not suffer extreme poverty as the UN defines it. Perhaps no one in America will simply starve to death. But let's not fool ourselves. First-world poverty still puts people at risk. "Poverty is a thief," says Michael Reich. "Poverty not only diminishes a person's life chances, it steals years from one's life."[30]

That 10 or 20 percent who were already on the edge? Many of them could soon find themselves pushed over it. Even with relief bills and paycheck protections, in the first months of lockdowns we started seeing stories of lines for food pantries stretching sometimes for miles. In the wealthiest country in human history.

DEATHS AND ILLNESS FROM DELAYS IN MEDICAL CARE

An NPR story in early May reported on a woman who "had the worst headache of her life," but put off treatment for fear of the coronavirus. As a result, she had multiple strokes and died of a "brain bleed." Her doctor thought her death was preventable.

The story was about the worrisome trend of patients avoiding emergency rooms when they had heart attacks and strokes. "Across the country," explained the president of the American College of Emergency Physicians, "ER volumes are down about 40% to 50%."[31] Over the whole country, "911 call volumes for strokes and heart attacks declined in March through early April." Were people having fewer heart attacks and strokes, or were they fearful of calling ambulances to take them to hospitals, which the press had portrayed as death traps?

Clinical stroke centers saw "an 'unprecedented' drop in stroke patients being treated, with decreases ranging from 50% to 70%." One doctor said he worried "it could be challenging to care for all the patients who eventually show up at hospitals in even worse shape after delaying care." Another doctor, a board president in L.A. of the American Heart Association, asked, "Are these people dying at home?"

After spending months feeding the panic, the press grew interested in this story about the unintended consequences of the panic. On May 25, Katie Hafner of the *New York Times* wrote about doctors trying and failing to get patients with serious problems to come in. Why? Panic about catching the coronavirus.

Hafner quoted a Brown University psychiatrist. "If you have anxiety and then you exacerbate that by watching the news and reading social media, that's where you get panicked," the professor explained. "And the rational, thinking parts of the brain stop functioning well when we're panicked."[32] You don't say.

Many folks avoided medical attention because of the panic. But government decrees also kept people from getting medical care. Authorities defined many "elective" medical procedures as inessential. And while "elective" may sound to most people like tummy tucks and facelifts, in fact it means procedures that patients have scheduled, as opposed to, say, getting a broken bone set during a trip to the emergency room. But of course, we schedule brain surgery, heart surgery, and cancer surgery, knee, hip, and back surgery. These life-saving surgeries were delayed, sometimes for months.

At first, we presume, these decrees against health care came from the model-induced fears that hospitals would be overrun with COVID-19 patients. You know, back when we were still trying to flatten the curve. Even then, authorities were foolishly prioritizing the treatment of the coronavirus over the treatment of hundreds of other deadly illnesses. Government was, in effect, rationing healthcare by fiat based on anticipated shortages. But the curve-flattening argument became obsolete in April when the shortages never came, and yet the restrictions continued. As a result, we've not only delayed life-saving treatments but also crippled our health-care system. In April alone, 1.4 million jobs were lost in that sector.[33]

Millions of people have suffered while waiting. Imagine needing hip surgery, suffering in pain for months while the hospital is half empty and your surgeon has had to furlough staff for lack of patients. Then multiply that a few million times to get some sense of the collective toll of these misguided policies.

And then there were the deaths. In Ontario, thirty-five patients died in March and April waiting for heart procedures.[34] A May 5 article at Medscape predicted that a lockdown lasting three months (until June) "could mean 80,000 missed cancer diagnoses."[35] We can't yet say how many "collateral" deaths from missed treatment there will be from the lockdowns. But they could outweigh the number of deaths from COVID-19 itself.

Scott Atlas, former chief of Neuroradiology at Stanford University Medical Center, has argued just that.[36] Atlas and colleagues have calculated that "the national lockdown is responsible for at least 700,000 lost years of life every month." The details are depressing:

> Here are the examples of missed health care on which we base our calculations: Emergency stroke evaluations are down 40 percent. Of the 650,000 cancer patients receiving chemotherapy in the United States, an estimated half are missing their treatments. Of the 150,000 new cancer cases typically discovered each month in the U.S., most—as elsewhere in the world—are not being diagnosed, and two-thirds to three-fourths of routine cancer screenings are not happening because of shutdown policies and fear among the population. Nearly 85 percent fewer living-donor transplants are occurring now, compared to the same period last year. In addition, more than half of childhood vaccinations are not being performed, setting up the potential of a massive future health disaster.[37]

While experts will debate exact numbers for the next several years, the numbers here are so large that we have no doubt that the lapse in care will end up costing many lives.

Wasted Goods

The U.S. supply chain is a wonder to behold. Most of us never even notice it. We take well-stocked grocery stores and restaurants for granted. We expect next-day delivery from Amazon, and usually get it. Many parts of the chain use just-in-time inventories, which cuts costs and waste.

Supply chains for groceries and online stores slowed during the lockdowns, but still worked miraculously well for months. Sure, toilet paper and hand sanitizer disappeared because of hoarding, but not for long. Weird things like chai tea became scarce. But stores were still well-stocked with fruit and vegetables, frozen and dry goods, pet food, and pretty much everything we needed.

In the restaurant sector, though, a catastrophe unfolded. We've mentioned the small businesses and millions of employees. But did you wonder what happened to all that *food*? You might have imagined that pork and eggs destined for diners got rerouted to Safeway and Costco. But that's not how it works, especially with perishable items. When millions of Americans quit eating out, that sent shockwaves back up the supply chain.

Americans typically get about 40 percent of their food not from the grocery store, but from restaurants—dine-in and takeout. Chicken or eggs or pork packaged and prepared for, say, Applebee's can't simply be sent to Safeway. Safeway has its own supply chain, with suppliers, trucks, scheduled deliveries, and so forth.

So what happened to all that restaurant-bound food in the lockdowns? Without income, the restaurants couldn't pay for it. So, they stopped placing orders, and before long, there were armies of growing hogs and chickens with no place to go. Farmers can't tell chickens to stop laying eggs and cows to stop producing milk. Cheese and butter can be stored, but there's only so much refrigeration space around. Within

weeks, farmers had to start dumping milk[38] and produce[39] and euthaniz-
ing animals.[40] One story in early May reported that farmers were killing
ten thousand pigs a day—in Minnesota alone.[41]

All this, while ever more Americans had less to eat.

CRIME

One of the most bizarre policy choices in the coronavirus panic was
blue states such as California (and blue zones in red states) furloughing
prisoners. Travis County (home to liberal Austin, Texas) released almost
six hundred felons. Among them were prisoners convicted of aggravated
assault, arson, attacking a peace officer, and human trafficking.[42] When
Texas governor Greg Abbott issued an executive order banning such
releases, the ACLU sued him.[43]

The *New York Post* reported that "at least 50 of the 1,500 inmates
cut loose amid fears of the spread of COVID-19 behind bars in recent
weeks have already landed back in jail—and in some cases were set free
yet again."[44] Ben Johnson offered a litany of such stories at The Stream.
"In New York City, burglaries are up 37% and murders have nearly
tripled," he wrote. "With only 10% of their usual commuters, the number of NYC subway robberies has risen 29%. In Seattle, burglaries have
spiked, nearly doubling since the stay-at-home order."[45]

Foreign fraudsters took advantage of the surge in unemployment
payments by stealing the identities of employed Americans and conning
state governments into covering bogus unemployment claims.[46] This
fraud is estimated to have added hundreds of millions of dollars to the
total taxpayer bill.

Reuters reported a rise in depraved landlords requiring sex from
tenants who, because of job losses, could not make rent. Accompanying
this has been a "rise in online adverts offering rent-free accommodation
in exchange for sexual favours."[47]

The most heartbreaking development, though, was like the famous
Sherlock Holmes story of the dog that did not bark. After the lockdowns

went into effect, reports of child abuse plummeted. But that didn't mean that child abuse had declined. Rather, the ways that authorities usually detect such abuse—warning signs reported by teachers, emergency room doctors, first responders—dried up. In March, states such as Massachusetts, Connecticut, and New Hampshire saw reported cases drop roughly in half overnight.[48] This at a time when stress and shelter-in-place orders almost surely meant more rather than less child abuse.

How many kids were not rescued from abuse because so many of the chances for detecting and stopping it were shut down? Some sources reported an increase in ER visits during the crisis for children with injuries, though these could have arisen from children simply being home and outside more and not in school.[49] Time will tell.

LOSS OF TRUST

What's the lesson of the story of the boy who cried wolf? It's not that wolves don't exist. It's that you shouldn't sound false alarms, lest people doubt you in a real emergency.

Health authorities across the world find themselves in the same predicament as the boy who didn't really see a wolf. Maybe this isn't all bad. We'd be lying if we said we mourn the loss of trust in the UN and WHO. The world might be a better place if the UN campus were turned into condos and the organization were replaced with a loose alliance of nations that value human rights. And it's unhealthy for a corrupt political entity such as WHO to have so much sway over global health. Science, like markets, does better when it's dispersed.

But what if we ever *do* have to deal with a truly historic pathogen? With the global army of boys crying wolf, how credible would WHO, the CDC, and so forth be in sounding the alarm? Who, outside the media, would take their word for it? People are bound to be far less docile the second time around, far less inclined to heed early warnings. Social media might fill the void, but is that a good solution?

Some companies cashed in on the boy's cry, and inspired paranoia in the process. Contact tracing became a fertile ground for dystopian tech.

It brought Apple and Google together for a joint project using Bluetooth technology to detect when people are near each other.[50] Both corporations assured us that they would protect our privacy. But with the surveillance system in place and everyone expected to give up their rights when the authorities say so, who can blame people for worrying?

It's not just the smartphone giants. AiRISTA Flow developed a device that could be worn around the neck. "When people come within six feet of each other for a period of time," a story in The Intercept explained, "the device makes an audible chirp and a record of the contact is made in the AiRISTA Flow software system."[51] This is an improvement over cattle branding, which is how the comings and goings of slaves in certain places were once tracked. But in those physically crueler days, there were at least no permanent databases that stored who you saw, where, and when.

GOVERNMENT EXPANSION AND TYRANNY

The response to the coronavirus surely marked the fastest and most sweeping growth of state power in history. States and cities seemed to compete for top prize in the Most Draconian Police Action.

Often these efforts had little to do with public safety. There was (and is) no evidence that the virus spreads easily outdoors. And yet around the country, cities closed golf courses. Ditto with boating and beaches. Maryland forbade families from boating together. Venice Beach in Los Angeles used tractors to fill a local skateboard park with beach sand. Aerial video of the tractors offered an arresting visual symbol of the petty tyrannies that had pockmarked the land of the free and the home of the brave within a few short weeks. California governor Gavin Newsom was trying to keep beaches closed as late as May, though by that point the public had started to rebel, and sheriffs of multiple counties refused to enforce the closures.[52]

Gretchen Whitmer, the governor of Michigan, didn't stop at pronouncing many businesses non-essential. She prevented the big-box stores that remained open from selling unapproved goods. One story highlighted the plight of a mother in Big Rapids, Michigan, who couldn't buy a car seat at a local Walmart because of the order.[53] "Everything I'm doing is trying to save your life," Whitmer insisted.[54] She may have been sincere in that. If so, she just has a very narrow view of life.

Tyranny is a perennial threat. Death by government was one of the leading causes of premature death in the twentieth century.[55] And, of course, tyranny harms even those it doesn't kill. Scan the Index of Economic Freedom, which ranks countries according to the amount of economic freedom they enjoy. The details are messy, but the overall pattern is unmistakable. At the top you'll find the freer and wealthier places that people risk their lives to get into—New Zealand, Australia, Switzerland, Canada, Taiwan, the U.S., and so forth. At the bottom, the poor and tyrannical places that people risk their lives to get out of—North Korea, Cuba, Venezuela, Zimbabwe. You get the picture.

"Emergencies," Friedrich Hayek argued, "have always been the pretext on which the safeguards of individual liberty have eroded." Even when government growth during a crisis doesn't end in tyranny, it's very hard to wind things back when the crisis is over. Bureaucracies habitually perpetuate and expand themselves, and the public, which might have opposed a program at first, comes to rely on it after it's in place.[56] That makes government growth a one-way ratchet.

The eight-hundred-page CARES Act involved all manner of economic meddling, but at least it was aimed at helping Americans who had lost their jobs. The arbitrary attacks on religious freedom were another thing entirely. Governors declared churches and places of worship nonessential, and churches closed their doors in service to the common good. But then the lockdowns went on and on and on, and the bias against churches became more obvious. In mid-May, for instance, Minnesota governor Tim Walz allowed tattoo parlors, malls, and even casinos to reopen, but not churches. Understandably, Catholics and Lutherans in the state protested. The archbishop of Minneapolis and St. Paul, Bernard Hebda, had finally had enough. He wrote the governor a short letter, explaining, "We feel compelled by pastoral need to provide our people with an opportunity to come together on Pentecost, before the Easter season concludes. We hope that the care with which we have prepared for a return to in-person worship will publicly manifest that we continue to share your goal of protecting lives and safeguarding the well-being of the community during this challenging time."[57]

Though the archbishop did not quote Benjamin Franklin, who was not a good Christian, we will: "Rebellion to tyrants is obedience to God." The archbishop's act of rebellion worked: the governor caved.[58]

What price do we put on freedom? How much pain or risk are we willing to endure to preserve it? How we answer that question may well determine the future.

A Grab Bag of Human Costs

We can't treat all the costs of the panic and lockdown at the length they deserve. But we should at least list some others:

- Disruption and loss of education from kindergarten through graduate school
- Missed worship and other religious services
- Unmeasurable anxiety, depression, loneliness, and anger[59]
- Escalating pornography use and addiction[60]
- Substance abuse and setbacks in recovery[61]
- Weight gain and fewer options for exercise[62]
- Lost lifetime experiences from canceled and altered weddings and funerals, and canceled vacations, graduation ceremonies, concerts, symphonies, ballets, musicals, plays, birthday parties, and sporting events[63]

No doubt there are more costs, but this chapter is already too depressing. We hope we've proved our point: the cost of the nationwide panic and the lockdowns was immense, and far beyond any benefit we could have hoped to achieve. It's certainly beyond any benefit we did achieve.

ARE WE ALREADY SEEING EXCESS DEATHS FROM THE LOCKDOWN?

We have argued that the lockdowns put in place to save lives from the coronavirus are bound to claim lives by the tens or hundreds of thousands. It may take years for some of these premature deaths—such as those resulting from lost medical care—to take place. But can we already see evidence of some excess deaths?

To answer this question, we first need to know how many deaths were caused by the coronavirus. You'd think we could get reliable numbers for this. After all, these figures were constantly in the headlines. Alas, even the official sources disagree, though the discrepancies are mostly small until we approach the current date. In Figure 10.1 we again see the weekly all-cause deaths. There is some uncertainty at the end of the figure because CDC advises that data can be adjusted up or down, (usually up), as many as eight weeks after the data are published.[64]

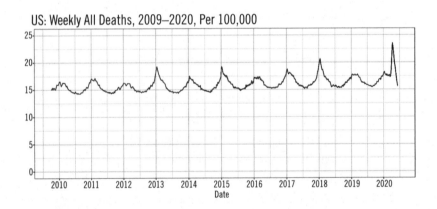

US: Weekly All Deaths, 2009–2020, Per 100,000

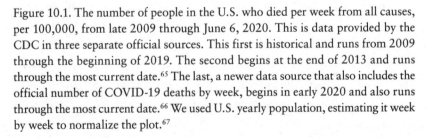

Figure 10.1. The number of people in the U.S. who died per week from all causes, per 100,000, from late 2009 through June 6, 2020. This is data provided by the CDC in three separate official sources. This first is historical and runs from 2009 through the beginning of 2019. The second begins at the end of 2013 and runs through the most current date.[65] The last, a newer data source that also includes the official number of COVID-19 deaths by week, begins in early 2020 and also runs through the most current date.[66] We used U.S. yearly population, estimating it week by week to normalize the plot.[67]

Deaths from all causes peak around January each year because of the flu and associated diseases including pneumonia. The varying height of the January spikes shows that some flu seasons are worse than others. As we saw in chapter 3, the 2017–2018 flu season was particularly brutal.

It's important to note the slow increase in the death rate from year to year. This is most likely due to an increase in the mean age as the huge Boomer generation makes its exit.

The prominent peak starting in March 2020 is due to the coronavirus. Flu-associated deaths, which normally peak in January, were low in this shorter-than-normal flu season, meaning there were fewer flu-associated deaths from pneumonia. This year, the coronavirus may have claimed some lives that a more dangerous flu strain would have claimed.

US: Weekly All Deaths, Late 2017–June 2020

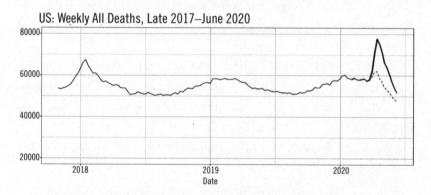

Figure 10.2. All-cause weekly deaths from late 2017 onwards, using two official sources of CDC data. The dashed line is the all-caused death minus the official COVID deaths, using the CDC's COVID death page. The line becomes thicker at the end because of slight discrepancies in the CDC sources.

Figure 10.2 shows the raw death numbers from all CDC sources. The 2017–2018 flu season produced a larger peak than the two flu seasons that followed. The highest peak, following the 2019–2020 flu season, is associated with the coronavirus pandemic. Let's see how closely associated. The dashed line shows all-cause deaths minus the official COVID-19 numbers—in other words, deaths by everything *but* the coronavirus.

In most years, deaths are on the way down by April. In 2020 they peaked a second time in that dashed line. If we accept the official numbers, then these unusual deaths have some other cause. Now it may be that these "extra" deaths are COVID-19 deaths somehow missed by all the people eager to classify deaths as coronavirus—though that seems unlikely. Or they might be genuine non-COVID deaths, as the CDC thinks.[68]

What caused the re-spike in non-COVID deaths? One possible culprit is the lockdowns themselves. Delayed treatment led to at least some deaths. Perhaps being cooped up inside also is harmful in itself. Lockdowns force the healthy and sick into tight quarters, enhancing the spread of all communicable diseases. At least in the United States, the lockdowns threw younger and healthier people out of work and forced them to stay home, sometimes with older, sickly relatives. Both lockdowns and fear forced people inside.

England and Wales had a harsher lockdown than the United States. Several American states never locked down at all, and even in some states with lockdowns, enforcement was not thorough, especially outside cities.

With that in mind, here are the all-caused weekly per capita deaths for England and Wales.

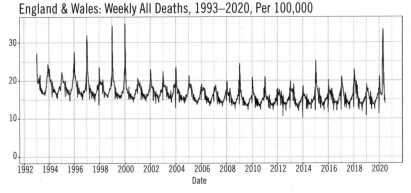

England & Wales: Weekly All Deaths, 1993–2020, Per 100,000

Figure 10.3. The all-cause weekly deaths from England and Wales, from 1993 to May 15, 2020. Office of National Statistics.[69]

It is clear from Figure 10.3 that the 2020 coronavirus peak was not as bad as the 1999–2000 flu year in England and Wales. The coronavirus about tied the 1998–1999 flu season. Remember, there were no lockdowns in those flu years. In Figure 10.4, the dashed line shows the difference between all-cause deaths and official COVID deaths.

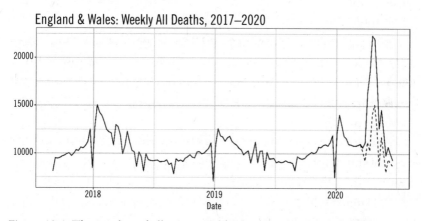

Figure 10.4. The number of all-cause weekly deaths in England and Wales from 2017 through June 19, 2020. The dashed line is the all-cause deaths minus the official COVID-19 deaths.

First, in many years there's a dip in reported deaths on or about December 25. Whether this is from people trying to eke out one last Christmas or because the bureaucracy shuts down for a week, we don't know. At any rate, the coronavirus peak in 2020 is obvious.

But so is the dashed line. It's much larger than in the United States, which means that England and Wales had more "extra" deaths from causes other than the coronavirus than we did. Again, we can't prove that lockdowns caused these extra deaths. But the skeptic is under the burden of proving, and not just hoping or assuming, that the coronavirus caused these deaths. This will be tough: after all, officials bent over backwards to attribute even suspected cases to the virus.

We are not the only ones to notice this strange and unexpected spike. A paper published May 13 by the *British Medical Journal* was entitled

"Covid-19: 'Staggering Number' of Extra Deaths in Community Is Not Explained by Covid-19."[70] It reported that "care homes and other community settings had had to deal with a 'staggering burden' of 30,000 more deaths than would normally be expected, as patients were moved out of hospitals that were anticipating high demand for beds." And, "Of those 30,000, only 10,000 have had covid-19 specified on the death certificate." These match our estimates from the spike.

The paper quotes epidemiologist David Leon: "Some of these deaths may not have occurred if people had got to hospital. How many is unclear. This issue needs urgent attention, and steps taken to ensure that those who would benefit from hospital treatment and care for other conditions can get it."

Whether or not lockdowns somewhere slowed the spread of the virus, we must judge the panic and the lockdowns by both successes and harms. The real costs of the panic and lockdowns, short and long term, vastly exceeded the benefits.

CHAPTER 11

LIFE, DEATH, AND THE PURSUIT OF HAPPINESS

We hold these truths to be self-evident, that all men are created equal, that they are endowed by their creator with certain unalienable rights, that among these are life, liberty, and the pursuit of happiness.

—*The Declaration of Independence*

Before the coronavirus crisis hit, American conservatives almost came to blows arguing about the "common good." One side avoided the term because they saw it as a euphemism for the nanny state—big-government progressivism in which a central power dictates everyone's life goals and movements, whether they like it or not. The other side defended it as a bulwark against the college libertarian's vision of the state as nothing more than a night watchman.

The Catechism of the Catholic Church defines the common good as "the sum total of social conditions which allow people, either as groups or as individuals, to reach their fulfillment more fully and more easily." In other words, at a minimum, the good of the commons or society as a whole must include the goods of individuals, families, neighborhoods, and church communities. And most people agree that government ought to protect those goods—or, at the very least, not subvert them.

In the panic over the pandemic, in contrast, authorities seemed to be guided by a narrow goal that no sane society would embrace: namely, prevent wherever possible every coronavirus casualty, no matter the cost in lives or fortune.

This was a deeply misguided goal. And it was in fatal conflict with the core principles of the American Experiment.

RIGHTS BEFORE RESULTS

In the United States we have always organized our political life around a set of principles that limits what authorities can and ought to do. These limiting principles trump any overarching societal goal. These principles are the "rights" enshrined in our Constitution. These rights prevent the majority from tyrannizing the minority. They keep Americans from holding people as expendable in pursuit of the greatest good for the greatest number. They stop citizens from treating their fellow citizens as mere means to their ends—however noble those ends may be.

Imagine, for instance, a fifty-year-old man named Harold doing life in prison for armed robbery. He has no friends or family or joy in his life, but he is healthy. He has two good kidneys, two good lungs, a heart, and a liver.

As it happens, there are six twelve-year-old children in a hospital nearby in desperate need of organ transplants. If we could just harvest Harold's organs and give them to the children, we could save the six innocent children with long futures ahead of them, in exchange for perhaps fifteen future years of Harold's dreary life. So, what keeps us from taking Harold's organs?

Sure, it would be first-degree murder, which suggests that it's a bad thing to do. But why is it bad? Because Harold has a right to his life. That right forbids others from harming him arbitrarily, whether for organ harvesting or any other reason. The fact that by killing Harold we could save the lives of six children and net far more life-years is beside the point. The good—saving the children—doesn't override the evil.

Harold has rights, and we have a corresponding duty to respect them.

Behind this notion of a right is a vision of human dignity and flourishing that, if you're an American at least, you likely believe even if you've never quite worked out the logic of it.

That vision inspired the founding of our nation and shaped the principles of our government. In the United States, the role of the government is to establish justice, protect the rights of citizens, promote the general welfare, preserve the blessings of liberty, and so forth. Basic police powers to protect us against harm from others are mostly exercised by the states. We rightly take it for granted that both federal and local governments will, at a minimum, recognize and protect our basic rights.

That's why it was so disturbing when, in the coronavirus crisis, government officials at every level disregarded Americans' basic rights—especially their rights to assembly and to the free exercise of religion. Even worse? Americans, in our panic, seemed ready to surrender those rights for safety.

We chose the extreme example of organ harvesting to appeal to your basic moral sense. Most of us recoil at the thought of invoking a "greater good" to justify murder, or even the nonlethal extraction of organs. At some level we know, even if we sometimes forget, that a just society does not pursue even worthy goals or maximize a single abstract good—such as safety or income equality—at the expense of our basic rights. Our government doesn't guarantee us happiness—only the right to pursue it. Much less can it guarantee perfect safety to us all. No one can live a risk-free life. And at some point, everyone dies. However we think about public health, we should not forget those two facts.

BUT WHAT ABOUT PUBLIC HEALTH?

Of course, we're not saying that the state has no role to play in public health. But public health officials left to their own devices are not likely to get the balance right. They're bound to maximize safety, to the neglect of other goods. In this way, they're like doctors who run every possible test on a patient. Looking for problems is a physician's job. Misdiagnosis could be malpractice. This makes them risk-averse and hypervigilant. But you, as a patient, have different aims. What you deem best for you, weighing costs and benefits, may not be what's best for the doctor who's treating you.

This is why putting medical specialists in charge of nations—or the whole globe—is asking for overly cautious and even oppressive policies. These experts tend to become fixated on the single malady in front of them, to the exclusion of any other concern. With tragic results for us in the United States—and every other country that followed the doctors' orders.

We offer, as Exhibit A, Dr. Ezekiel Emanuel, oncologist, bioethicist, and one-time public health guru under President Obama. Probably for shock value, news outlets quoted him in April 2020 saying that the whole country must be locked down for twelve to eighteen months until there was a vaccine: "Realistically, COVID-19 will be here for the next 18 months or more. We will not be able to return to normalcy until we find a vaccine or effective medications," he said. "I know that's dreadful news to hear. How are people supposed to find work if this goes on in some form for a year and a half? Is all that economic pain worth trying to stop COVID-19? The truth is we have no choice."[1]

The doctor was wrong. There is always a choice. We could have gone on with our lives, just as people did during the swine flu, the Asian flu, the Hong Kong flu, and on and on. Failing that, at least we could have pivoted as soon as we saw that the coronavirus was not as deadly as predicted.

Why couldn't Emanuel see this? For the same reason Exhibit B, presidential advisor Anthony Fauci, said, "I don't think we should ever shake hands ever again, to be honest with you. Not only would it be good to prevent coronavirus disease; it probably would decrease instances of influenza dramatically in this country."[2] This from the man *The New Yorker* called "America's Doctor."[3]

In mid-May, Fauci spoke to a Senate health committee about the dangers of reopening schools and warned governors of "needless suffering and death" if we re-opened states "prematurely." Prematurely, compared to what? The word implies a fixed end date, like a due date during a pregnancy. But Fauci promised no end date to the madness.

Why do doctors like Emanuel and Fauci say such things? Because they're in the grip of a single goal. Public health officials tend to think in bulk, to focus on the quantity of abstract life protected in the near term, rather than the quality of actual lives lived over the long term. Imagine, for instance, what might happen if a risk-averse public health expert who had spent 30 years obsessing over traffic deaths could dictate the driving choices of 330 million Americans, or 8 billion humans. It wouldn't be pretty.

The problem is not expertise. We all benefit from experts. The problem is the *tyranny* of experts—when their narrow, professionally biased thinking dictates policy for everyone. In a sane world, the media would grasp that experts such as Emanuel and Fauci offer one narrow take on a vast and complex problem, and that while we shouldn't ignore them, we shouldn't idolize them either.

Regrettably, the press weaponized Fauci against President Trump and other politicians who challenged the wisdom of an indefinite shutdown. The headlines reporting on Fauci's May testimony before a Senate committee—when Senator (Dr.) Rand Paul had the temerity to tell him, "You're not the end-all"—were predictable: "Trump's Push to Reopen Schools Clashes with Fauci's Call for Caution"; "Fauci Warns of Colossal, Deadly Mistake. Will Trump Listen?"; "Fauci Warns: More Death, Econ Damage If US Reopens Too Fast."[4]

Of course, Fauci has no expertise in economics, and even his health advice had changed over the course of the winter and spring. As Steve Deace noted on May 14,

> In January, Fauci did an interview in his native NYC saying coronavirus was just another flu. In February, he wrote virtually the same in the *New England Journal of Medicine*. In March, he said Americans don't need to be walking

around wearing masks. Then later in March he told Congress this would kill 10 times more people than the flu. He signed up to lockdown the country based on the disgraced Imperial College Model in March, too. In April, he sentenced us to further lockdown based on the always wrong IHME model. Later in April he said he wasn't sure we could trust the models. Now in May he's not sure we can send the kids back to school this fall, a linchpin to reopening the country, despite the fact kids are returning to school in China, Japan, Switzerland, Iceland, Norway, Denmark, France, Israel, and Sweden.

So how do you know which Fauci to worship? Your demigod sure does change his mind a lot.[5]

No matter. The press had elevated Fauci and other specialists to the status of infallible oracles—whose most recent pronouncements erased whatever they'd said the day before—and dared governors and presidents to challenge them.

But challenge them we must.

SAFETY THIRD

What should be the goal of public health policy? It can't simply be to reduce the number of deaths. After all, when all is said and done, the number of death certificates always equals the number of birth certificates. We can delay death, sometimes for decades, but we can't abolish it.

Indeed, if our main national goal was to reduce the number of deaths, then we should reduce the number of births. As soon as the human race goes the way of the dodo bird, we've met our goal!

That can't be right. We may disagree on the ultimate purpose of our lives, but most of us still agree that life is worth living even though it ends in death.

And we accept that there's an average life expectancy. We also agree that it's good to avert death and save life, as much as we can, consistent with our other goals. But reducing an abstract number of deaths can't be the goal of our public policy.

What makes more sense is to count the years that are lost to premature death and try to save them, insofar as this is consistent with our other goals. Obviously, losing one day of your life is less costly than losing a month, or a year, or a decade. The more of your life you lose, the less chance you have to pursue happiness. We shouldn't compare the value of one person's life to another. Each person is unique and unrepeatable. That's why we recoil in horror at the organ-harvesting story. Still, the death of nine-year-old Billy in a car wreck is tragic in a way that Billy's death at age ninety-nine from natural causes isn't. In the second case, he had the chance to live a full life. In the first case, he would not have. And in the case of Billy Graham, he not only had a chance to live a full life. He did.

As we explained in chapter 10, economists can figure out (roughly) how much we would be willing to spend to reduce the risk of losing a year of our lives by studying how much we spend (collectively) on fire alarms, airbags, and the like. Right now in the United States, that number is around $150,000. Using that figure, we can measure the costs of premature deaths in terms of a quantity known as "years of life lost."

Of course, we don't know, ahead of time, how long anyone will live. If Emma dies in a construction accident when she's thirty-two, how many years did she lose? That is, how long would she have lived otherwise? We can't know. So, for health policy questions, we use averages. As the Organization for Economic Co-operation and Development explains, we can calculate years of life lost by "summing up deaths occurring at each age and multiplying this with the number of remaining years to live up to a selected age limit."[6] This limit is usually around average life expectancy at birth, about seventy years.[7]

Again, the point is not to put a price on every life, or to say that your value declines with age. The point is to get a grasp of how much deadly risk we freely tolerate in living our lives. That is, how do we as a society weigh the risk of death, injury, and the like against other ends we pursue? This is what we do for other risks, rather than pursuing safety at all costs.[8]

With that in mind, we can use age-at-death statistics published by the CDC[9] to calculate the cost of the coronavirus in years of life lost. As of May 28, 2020, this comes out to just over 400,000 years in the U.S. That's a lot of life, to be sure. But for perspective, we need to compare it to a more familiar risk. When we do the same calculation on U.S. traffic deaths in 2017,[10] we find that these caused about three times as many years of life to be lost—over 1.2 million. Although collisions killed about half as many people as the coronavirus—just over 40,000 as compared to just over 80,000 on one estimate—the mean age of people killed on the roads was much younger—45 years compared to 76 years.

In other words, for generations we have accepted a higher annual loss of years from driving. We've done this because we valued our freedom to travel by road more than we valued the 1.2 million years of life we give up for this freedom. And we weren't crazy to do so. Think about it. When you saw the scary films of fatal crashes in drivers' education class as a teenager, did you vow never to travel by car? Or were you, instead, motivated to drive carefully so as to enjoy the freedom while reducing the risks? Most of us refused to let fear rob us of that freedom. Indeed, the point of the films was not to get us all to cower in our bedrooms until death takes us or the world ends. The point was to show us, as young drivers, the real dangers so we wouldn't take stupid risks.

Parents of young drivers have to risk losing their children to see them become responsible adults. That's the noble intent of all good parents. When parents do lose a child, the grief is immense. But no one thinks it would be better if we kept all teenagers locked in the basement, lest they have a car wreck. Life is for living, not merely for preserving.

Safety is rarely our main goal. For most ventures, your first goal is to do something. For instance, you get in the car to drive to work. Safety is important, but if it were your primary goal, you wouldn't get in the car. Mike Rowe often reminded viewers of this in his show *Dirty Jobs*. He even started talking about "Safety Third" in response to the ever-present OSHA posters in workplaces he visited.[11] Safety should be a high priority, but not *the* priority—not if you want to do a job, have a family, and live a life.

This is one reason the one-size-fits-all policies made no sense. There's a vast difference between a disease that kills indiscriminately—the old and the young, the healthy and the infirm—and a disease that mostly causes or contributes to the deaths of people near the end of their lives. It's the difference between losing 60 percent of your life and 2 percent, given that we all lose our lives in the end. No doubt this was what Texas lieutenant governor Dan Patrick meant when he said that "there are more important things than living…saving this country for my children and grandchildren.… I don't want to die, nobody wants to die, but man, we got to take some risks and…get this country back up and running."[12]

Of course, the press portrayed this as callous indifference toward the elderly—even though Patrick was referring to self-sacrifice. The point is not that we should sacrifice the lives of the old and frail for the young and healthy. We shouldn't. Rather, as a matter of public health, we should make sure that the costs of our interventions don't vastly exceed the benefits. Acting as if the virus was of equal danger to everyone, as if everyone's risk assessment should be the same—was bound to ensure the opposite.

Measuring the cost in life years gives us a way to take into account how we balance risk against other goods in real life. If a policy that saves one net life year costs far less than $150,000 and doesn't violate basic rights, then it's likely worth it. If it costs $10 million, that's a strong sign that it's a bad policy. It will probably cost more life years elsewhere and may involve injustice on top of that.[13] Economists are just starting to put a price tag in life years on the lockdowns, but one optimistic estimate put it at $700,000 per month, or $1.5 million by mid-June 2020. Whatever the total is, it will surely be much higher than that.[14]

We can now see how foolish it was to impose a quarantine on most of the population, at great cost. COVID-19 is far more deadly to the old and infirm, who are also least likely to work or be in school. So, obviously, we should have channeled resources to protecting them, rather than overriding everyone's basic rights, forcing young children inside, shutting down businesses, emptying hospitals, and setting up thousands of hospital beds that no one needed. We chose great pain for little or no gain.

The predictable refrain, of course, is that the pandemic would have claimed far more lives without the lockdown. But as we have seen, the evidence strongly suggests otherwise. We opted for a public health response that may have saved us nothing and will cost us hugely in life years. We'll spend the next several years coming to terms with the fact that we and our leaders profoundly misjudged both the benefits and the costs of lockdowns.

We recognize that choices in a crisis are hard to make. No one intended for more lives to be lost than gained, but that seems to be what happened. We found ourselves on that unintended course because we chose to respond to a worst-case scenario, just to be on the "safe" side.

Could we have done better? Yes. That's the subject of the next chapter.

CHAPTER 12

THROUGH A GLASS DARKLY: BALANCING COSTS WITH BENEFITS WHEN WE DON'T KNOW THE FUTURE

There are no solutions; there are only trade-offs.

—*Thomas Sowell*[1]

The original stated goal of the lockdown was simple: to "flatten the curve." In other words, to slow the rate of infection, thereby lowering the number of people sick with COVID-19 at any one time, to avoid overwhelming the hospitals. But as we have seen, it soon became clear that hospitals were in no risk of being overwhelmed. The fear of hospital overflows was based on the blind models that had also forecast millions of deaths. Both forecasts were badly wrong.

But by the time that became clear, elementary school students had been sent home, restaurants shuttered, Major League Baseball cancelled, and on and on and on. It seems it was too much for the powers that be to adjust to the facts. Instead, they kept moving the goalposts. Now the lockdown was about stopping the spread of the virus. And it wouldn't end after two weeks, or thirty days. Now we'd have to wait for summer, widespread testing, contact tracing, or even a vaccine. Which might not arrive until after the November election.[2] How convenient.

The value of quarantining healthy people at home was unclear, beyond a vague claim that we were saving lives.

Of course, mere mortals can't weigh every cost and benefit of every action and assign them all probabilities. But we should at least weigh the purported benefits against the costs we can anticipate, taking into account the likelihood of both. In other words, before we embrace a second and third wave of shutdowns, we should do what we didn't do before opting for the original lockdown.

JUST ONE LIFE: WEIGHING COSTS AND BENEFITS

At the height of the coronavirus crisis, New York governor Andrew Cuomo said that "if everything we do saves just one life, I'll be happy." (This is the guy who a year earlier had signed a law that removed abortion from New York's criminal code and made it legal for any reason up until birth, but that's another matter.) He was perhaps invoking the principle that you can't put a price on human life. To quote the Declaration once again, we are all "created equal and endowed by our Creator with unalienable rights," including the right to life. Our value comes not from our stock market portfolio, our popularity, or our looks, but from the fact that we are, each of us, made in the image of God. In that sense, each of us has infinite worth.

But Cuomo was misstating the problem we faced, by assuming that lives were on one side poised against money, time, and convenience on the other. In reality, there are economic costs but also risks to lives on all sides because we don't have infinite wealth, infinite time, and perfect safety. Wealth, time, and safety are all scarce resources. We have to make choices, and every choice involves a trade-off. Anyone who doesn't grasp this is not equipped for political leadership. Governing is all about making tough choices.

As we have seen, the infinite worth of every person doesn't mean we should spend an infinite amount to prevent one death, or even spend all the finite wealth of the world to do so. Why? For one thing, because we would lose far more lives than we would save. If we literally spent all the wealth of the world to save one person's life, everyone else would starve to death.

During the height of the panic, CNN ran an "analysis" slamming critics of the shutdown. The piece, boosted by Apple News, was entitled, "The Dangerous Morality behind the 'Open It Up' Movement." What is that dangerous morality? Well, according to the article it's utilitarianism, which the reporter defined as "letting a minority suffer so that the majority may benefit."[3]

Oddly, the piece didn't cite a single conservative utilitarian. And the critic of the "open it up" movement it cited favorably—bioethicist Anita Allen, who served on President Obama's bioethics committee—is a staunch advocate of abortion rights. Again, another subject, but one that often exposes moral inconsistency. Our argument against panic and lockdowns doesn't hinge *at all* on letting a minority suffer for the good of the majority. (If that's not clear, re-read chapter 11.)

The choice isn't between letting some people get killed or preventing their deaths by killing other people. Rather, we want to make sure that, as a matter of public policy, our response matches the risk involved, because either inaction or overreaction could lead to more deaths and harm.

We all accept trade-offs and take calculated risks. You can always reduce your risk of something. Avoiding some risks—some costs—means you incur other costs. If you're too risk-averse, you will bear the cost of missing out on life, along with the health costs of anxiety and torpor. Most of us would rather take our chances with cars and outside air.

No thinking person treats safety as the only good worth having. No thinking society does either. "Doing everything we can to save just one life" would justify banning all forms of travel, all sports, most recreation, all but the most sterile and bland foods, all potential allergens, and all person-to-person contact, including handshakes. Such a society would be a dystopian police state whose subjects spend all their time planning their escape.

These points should be obvious to every adult. Regrettably, they seem not to be. Early efforts to raise alarm about the huge costs of the public and government response to the coronavirus were met with outrage. What sort of heartless brute weighs dollars and cents against human lives?! The dilemma was reduced to a mental cartoon: scales with stacks of cash on one side, and old folks on the other. As Scott Adams put it on Twitter (tongue in cheek), "Tell me how many grandmas you would end to get back to work."

In fact, the tradeoff was never between filthy lucre and human lives. It was between lives harmed or lost from the viral outbreak and lives harmed or lost from our efforts to mitigate it. As we saw earlier, this includes what we did to our institutions, families, schools, businesses, churches, cities, states, countries, markets, and minds. Forecasts of death that were off by a factor of thirty were bound to summon a cure far worse than the disease. As Bruce Schneier has noted, "Security is all about tradeoffs, but when the stakes are considered infinitely high, the whole equation gets thrown out of kilter."

In the real world, every action has some cost, and so some risk—including what economists call "opportunity costs." If you choose to spend your lunch hour at McDonalds, you've ruled out eating at Arby's, going to the gym, and taking a nap. So, you incur the cost in dollars of your Big Mac and fries, but you also incur the cost of not doing the other things you could have done with that time and money.

In the same way, there are trade-offs, and opportunity costs, both to accepting and to avoiding risk. This side of glory, there's no such thing as zero risk—only more or less risk. So, the question we should be asking about any recommended response: Do the likely gains outweigh the costs—at least the ones we can foresee?

For instance, for years, the American Academy of Pediatrics has called on the Federal Aviation Administration (FAA) to mandate that infants under two be belted on commercial flights.[4] That sounds like a no-brainer. It's safer to wear a seat belt when flying on a plane because of the risk of turbulence. Thus, infants should wear seat belts. End of argument.

So why does the FAA allow parents to hold young infants on their laps without seat belts? Do they hate babies? No. They've just thought through the unintended effects of mandating seat belts (and so extra seats) for infants. In 2004, forty-three thousand people died on U.S. highways, but only thirteen on commercial flights.[5] If the FAA were to mandate that young children have their own seats, the added cost of flying would make driving more attractive to young families on tight budgets. And driving is clearly more dangerous.

Even the American Academy of Pediatrics admits that "the risk of death or serious injury in an aircraft is exceedingly small." In fact, from 1981 to 1997, there were only *three* reported deaths from injuries due to turbulence on commercial flights.[6] So why does the group still lobby for restraints for infants? Simple: it takes a very narrow view of risk.

After all, the infant in a lap in row eighteen is at greater risk than the infant buckled in a seat in row nineteen. So, for infants on flights, seats are better than laps. But the picture changes if a policy pushes infants from flights to freeways. Thus, the FAA only urges but does not mandate seats for infants.

The coronavirus presented us with this sort of Sophie's Choice: death to the left and death to the right. Of course, no one should opt to save ten people if a hundred others would be killed in the process. But usually the dilemma isn't so obvious, since it involves a seen and an unseen group. We feel much more strongly about people we can see than people we can't see. That's only natural. But it can lead to dreadful policies.

Highlighting unintended consequences is perhaps the greatest gift economics has given to humanity. "There is only one difference between a bad economist and a good one," wrote French economist Frédéric Bastiat. "The bad economist confines himself to the *visible* effect; the good economist takes into account both the effect that can be seen and those effects that must be *foreseen*." He explains: "Yet this difference is tremendous; for it almost always happens that when the immediate consequence is favorable, the later consequences are disastrous, and vice versa. Whence it follows that the bad economist pursues a small present good that will be followed by a great evil to come, while the good economist pursues a great good to come, at the risk of a small present evil."[7] Alas, the good economist has limited use in politics. Politicians tend to focus on the visible—the seen—since the unseen does little to help their prospects for reelection.

That logic holds in the response to a pandemic. Politicians must respond, and be seen responding, to the visible effects. It's natural to focus on reducing deaths from illness because the connection is so manifest. The people who died today were ill yesterday. Collateral casualties from measures like lockdowns are less visible because they're various and sundry and they take time, maybe even years, to come to pass. Presidents and prime ministers will tend to focus more on visible short-term deaths and disasters than long-term ones, even if there are far more of the latter than the former.

The choice was never going to be simple. From what we knew at the outset, forcing people to stay at home might do little good. Worse, it might even cause deaths, especially if high-risk and low-risk people huddled together.[8] Quarantining low-risk groups could cause deaths by delaying herd immunity and wasting resources. A recession could cause deaths from delays in health care and increased poverty. Even Governor Andrew Cuomo finally admitted that in early May: "There's a cost of staying closed, no doubt—economic cost, personal cost. There's also a cost of reopening quickly. Either option has a cost."[9]

But the details are complex. In wealthy countries, for instance, net deaths may actually drop during recessions.[10] Yes, suicides go up, but, weirdly, fewer total people die. Perhaps people travel less and take fewer risks. Indeed, one of the first effects of the great American lockdown was to reduce deadly car accidents.[11] At some point down the curve of economic ruin, though, that trend of fewer deaths will reverse as poverty kills more and more people. But a one-point drop in GDP need not add net deaths to the ledger.

All this is to say: to mount the right response, we needed to know the real risk we were facing. Short of that, we needed a way to decide without knowing. With the pandemic, as in life, none of us knew enough to foresee every outcome of every choice. All decision-makers, whether in local, state, or national governments, had to figure out what to do in the context of uncertainty.

WHEN YOU DON'T KNOW THE RISK

As it happens, there's a science called decision theory devoted to this very problem. It's an inexact science, in its infancy, and it can only help answer the simplest of questions. Still, there's some wisdom in it.

The theory offers three tactics for dealing with problems. The first and simplest is *Leave It Alone*. Don't worry about the problem and assume it will go away on its own. In one *Peanuts* cartoon, this was Charlie Brown's policy. "If you have some problem in your life," Linus asked Charlie, "do you believe you should try to solve it right away or think about it for a while?"

"Oh, think about it, by all means! I believe you should think about it for a while," Charlie answered.

"To give yourself time to do the right thing about the problem?"

"No," Charlie explained, "to give it time to go away!"

For some threats, that's the right choice. It's what the American government first did after learning about the coronavirus events unfolding in Asia in December 2019.

The second tactic is *One Step at A Time*. This is the sober approach. You gather relevant information, analyze it, then use it to figure out how likely this or that outcome is and what actions are within your power, given the options, and you weigh the costs and benefits you can anticipate. Then, you choose. If you get new data that points, say, north rather than south, you pivot northward. Taiwan and Singapore took this approach with the coronavirus.

The last approach, favored by American leaders, is the opposite of *Leave It Alone*. It's called *PANIC*. In politics, this tactic results in a look-at-me virtue-signaling arms race, with leaders trying to best each other in showing their commitment to the problem. In real-life emergencies, *Leave It Alone* is almost always followed by *PANIC*. Leaders worry that, since *Leave It Alone* didn't calm nerves, the press and the public will see *One Step at A Time* as too tepid. So they lurch to the other extreme and do too much.

Two different breeds of politicians adopt the *PANIC* approach, out of two different mindsets. The first is the grifter, the politician who uses the emergency to inflate his or her power. This kind of politician never lets a good crisis go to waste. Good crises are hard to find. That's why grifters do all they can to juice events to make them look worse than they are. Journalists often share this mindset.

The second mindset, far more common than the first, fully embraces worst-case-scenario thinking. Worrying about the worst that could happen drives much of our politics and public health decisions.

This mindset is common enough to have a name. It's called *the precautionary principle*.

Your Worst Nightmare

Early in 2020 a journalist named Ferris Jabr tried to calm an already growing panic. "None of this is to belittle what is happening," he wrote of the crisis developing in Wuhan. "The outbreak in China is a genuine public health emergency. But the essential data are still being collected and assessed. Sweeping and alarmist claims about unprecedented global threat are neither warranted nor helpful."

Nassim Taleb, author of the bestselling book *The Black Swan* and other works on decision-making, was having none of this. He dismissed Jabr as "Another ignorant journalist dealing with risk matters. Irresponsible."[12] Taleb preferred panic.

He was so incensed by the lack of panic that he and a number of co-authors wrote a brief paper to set the public straight.[13] They said that with the coronavirus "we are dealing with an extreme fat-tailed process." What does that mean? If you think of a standard bell curve as representing a common statistical distribution, the long tapering edges are referred to as *tails*. They're thin because extreme cases on either side are much rarer than cases in the middle. But in some situations, the extremes aren't so rare. The distributions for these can be called "fat-tailed."

Taleb's point was that the ease with which we now travel hither and yon changes the risk calculation for pandemics since extreme outcomes are much less rare than they used to be. "This means that expectations of the extent of harm are underestimates both because events are inherently fat-tailed, and because the tail is becoming fatter as connectivity increases."

It's true that greater connectivity will make pandemics occur more often. But Taleb is conflating the consequences of events with their chances. Rare events need not have greater consequences. If you throw a dozen pennies in the air and they all land heads up, we have a rare event all right, but who cares? The opposite is also true: frequent events can be consequential. Tornadoes hit the ground by the hundreds every year in the United States, often killing people and destroying property.

A more connected world makes infections spread across the globe more easily, but it's not clear this leads to worse consequences. It also helps us distribute resources better during pandemics, and it may even speed up herd immunity.

This brings us back to the precautionary principle—the idea that we should always prepare for the worst. Here's a paragraph from Taleb's paper: "Properties of the virus that are uncertain will have substantial impact on whether policies implemented are effective. For instance, whether contagious asymptomatic carriers exist. These uncertainties make it unclear whether measures such as temperature screening at major ports will have the desired impact. Practically all the uncertainty tends to make the problem potentially worse, not better, as these processes are convex to uncertainty."

This last point is wrong. There are plenty of unknown things, including *unknown* unknowns, which we can't even list as uncertainties because we haven't thought of them.[14] At the start of any crisis we stand on a beach, looking out at a sea of uncertainties, shrouded in a mist of mysteries. That doesn't mean all unknowns are bad. What we don't know could also be good, or benign. To assume that what we don't know must be *bad* is one of the precautionary principle's main panic-inducing fallacies.

PRECAUTION DECONSTRUCTED

Among the most quoted statements of the precautionary principle came from a 1998 conference at Wingspread, a famous Frank Lloyd Wright house in Wisconsin: "When an activity raises threats of harm to human health or the environment, precautionary measures should be taken even if some cause and effect relationships are not fully established scientifically. In this context the proponent of an activity, rather than the public, should bear the burden of proof."[15]

This makes perfect sense. A company wants to develop a genetically modified grain. The food made from the grain might cause harm. The burden is on the company to show otherwise.

With technology, the precautionary principle is commonsensical. Don't play God. But the same precautionary principle can go badly wrong when people try to apply it to natural dangers like pandemics. Assuming there was no evil scheme behind the coronavirus, there was no human choice to be made at the outset. No one weighed the risk of the pandemic and found it acceptable. It happened naturally, we presume. It was an act of God.

As we have seen, no one really knew what we were dealing with at first. Modelers tried to save the day with their predictions—which turned out to be little more than wild guesses. With the help of the press, it was easy to imagine the dreadful horrors. Some respected agencies suggested a coronavirus pandemic would kill tens of millions of people across the planet.[16]

Here's where the precautionary principle gets twisted from "Don't play God" to "trust me—I'm a god." By sleight of hand, the experts become oracles: to doubt their advice is to take foolish risks. The experts become gods, and any mere mortal who questions them is therefore *playing* god. Only in this light could lockdowns cease to be risks that carry a burden of proof. Instead, the skeptics who doubt them must bear that burden.

This inverted precautionary principle gives the experts license to imagine the worst-case scenario and then to agitate the government and the public to safeguard against this worst case. The mere chance that a disaster might happen is enough to justify any and all recommendations from the divine experts.

Having dispensed with probability, the experts concern themselves only with how bad the worst case would be. The zombie apocalypse is not likely, by any evidence we know of. Yet if it did happen, we would all die. There's no greater mortal cost.

Not to worry. The experts will hatch a plan to protect us, and considering the stakes, we would be fools not to do whatever they say. Only a psychopath would stand in their way.

Sound over-the-top? Nassim Taleb and his co-authors used just that word in describing the coronavirus risk: "Under such conditions it becomes selfish, even psychopathic, to act according to what is called 'rational' behavior—to make one's own immediate rankings of risk conflict with those of society, even generate risks for society. This is similar to other tragedies of the common, except that there is life and death." The quotation is from Taleb and Norman's one-page paper, "Ethics of Precaution: Individual and Systemic Risk,"[17] published in March 2020.

They also said, "Assume a risk of a multiplicative viral epidemic, still in its early stages. The risk for an individual to catch the virus is very low, lower than other ailments. It is therefore 'irrational' to panic (react immediately and as a priority). But if she or he does not panic and act in an ultra-conservative manner, they will contribute to the spread of the virus and it will become a severe source of systemic harm. Hence one must 'panic' individually (i.e., produce what seems to be an exaggerated response) in order to avoid systemic problems, even where the immediate individual payoff does not appear to warrant it."

Taleb and his co-author were arguing from the worst-case scenario, with no serious attention to the probabilities. The principle they articulate here could lead us to conclude that we should "panic and act in an ultra-conservative manner" in response to any and every conceivable threat, however unlikely. In fact, no one behaves that way. We weigh not only the severity but also the likelihood of the threats we face. And for good reason: we must husband our limited resources to meet the dangers that really threaten us.

The worst-case "multiplicative viral epidemic" comes much closer to the zombie apocalypse than the coronavirus has. In the zombie apocalypse everyone is at risk. Once bit, you must pass on the zombie cootie by biting others. For the coronavirus, not everybody was at risk of serious harm, and not everybody who got infected would pass it on. Which is normal in viral outbreaks and should have been expected.

Taleb and Norman fretted about the chance that the coronavirus could cause a "severe societal breakdown." Yet their imaginations failed them. They didn't foresee that the panic-induced cure would turn out to be worse than the disease.

CHAPTER 13

Who Got It Right?

A good example has twice the value of good advice.

—*Attributed to Albert Schweitzer*

Happily, there were a few countries and states that resisted the planetary panic. They offer a picture of what the rest of us could have done. And what we should do next time. For, like it or not, there will be a next time.

Made in Taiwan

As of June 1, 2020, seven people in Taiwan had died from the coronavirus. They counted 442 total cases of the disease, most of them in travelers coming there from abroad; fewer than half the cases were transmitted person to person in the country. Perhaps because of their traditional mistrust of China, Taiwan was one of the few countries that recognized the infection for what it was early on, and how it could be transmitted from person to person.[1]

The population of the country is a little under twenty-four million. Most of the people live in three large, sprawling metropolitan areas.

Taiwan never locked down, and never closed businesses. Schools never closed, though they delayed opening until February.[2] The government did issue periodic warnings about large gatherings, but never forbade them.[3] It asked the Catholic Church to limit large masses and other large assemblies. The bishops responded with a rolling church closing; by mid-March all public masses were canceled.[4] Buddhist temples remained open. Baseball, the most popular sport in the country, opened its season in April, albeit with robot and cardboard cutout "fans" at first. Fans were allowed back in limited numbers in mid-May.[5]

By any measure, this modern country, with more than twice as many people as Sweden or Belgium, did better than most others.

What did authorities do? They restricted travel to and from certain areas in China very early on, in January.[6] Taiwan kept a list of countries it considered higher risk, such as Iran and Italy. Early in March, people from these countries arriving at Taiwan airports had to go into a fourteen-day quarantine, either in their homes or designated hotels.[7] These people had to check in, via text messages, with the Taiwan CDC. Anybody showing symptoms could call a number and get treatment.[8]

One of us (William Briggs) happened to travel to Taiwan from New York City on business in early March. The only inconvenience I encountered was a three-hour wait inside the airport to fill out paperwork. The self-health check was no burden whatsoever. It was a piece of paper on which I could answer "Y" or "N" to whether I had a fever.

I could, and did, go anywhere I liked. I had been to Taiwan before, and the only change I noticed was more masks. There may have been fewer people going out to eat. Nowhere I went was closed. I was also in Singapore, Thailand, and Vietnam in January at the start of the crisis. The Asian media, like the Western media later, was full of COVID coverage, but it wasn't all worst-case scenario.

Late in March, travel to Taiwan was further restricted to citizens, diplomats, people on business, and the like.[9] To make that restriction less burdensome, the Taiwanese government allowed visitors to extend their visas. Flights off the island were scarce. Those to New York City would be posted, and then often cancelled—likely the result of American restrictions.

Travelers from certain other areas, and not just New York, that were deemed of moderate but not high risk, also faced fourteen days of self-health management. Like me, these people were free to travel anywhere. They just had to wear a mask while in public and check in with the CDC daily by responding to a text message.[10]

The Taiwanese are used to wearing masks. They consider it rude not to wear one if you're sick. Around flu season, masks are extremely common. They're not uncommon at other times of the year, either, such as when pollution is high.

There's a slightly more than healthy respect for disease transmission in Taiwan, an attitude that sometimes borders on paranoia. Few are immune to the media's haranguing. The country had been stung by SARS in 2003.

According to one paper by Taiwanese researchers, in the SARS outbreak, "346 SARS cases were officially confirmed in Taiwan, among which were 37 direct SARS deaths (cause of death was recorded as SARS) and 36 SARS-related deaths (cause of death was not directly attributed to SARS) as reported by the World Health Organization (WHO)."[11]

Even with these low numbers, more than 150,000 were quarantined in an effort to stop the spread of the disease. Did it work? Apparently not. The paper said, "The total number of confirmed SARS case-patients in Taiwan by the end of December 2004 was 480, of which 24 had been quarantined previously." It proved impossible to quarantine everyone who had been exposed. The virus seemed indifferent to the effort. The country learned that lesson and decided against aggressive quarantine for the coronavirus.

They took other measures, though. In mid-April, even as case numbers and deaths dropped, authorities mandated masks on public transportation, and later in banks and post offices.[12] They required masks in some larger businesses at the same time, even though daily new cases were already at or near zero, with only one new death in early May.

Early on, most large offices and other public buildings checked temperatures of entrants, often passively using infrared cameras or using handheld "gun" thermometers. Hand-sanitizer dispensers were ubiquitous. Some stores required "social distancing," placing markers where patrons could stand, as in the United States.[13] The rule was 1.5 meters between people, or about 5 feet.

Did these modest measures do anything? Who knows? What we do know is that the measures were modest. Taiwan did not shut down normal life and commerce, and the media there did not induce widespread panic, as in the United States. The country's CDC calmly announced every new measure as if it were reading a stock ticker.

Perhaps some measures, such as restricting travel from China, did some good: the virus never really got a foothold. At the very least, Taiwan proved it could manage a pandemic without a shutdown. Those claiming lockdowns are essential must explain how the country did so well without them.

Taiwan played a role in the global politics of the pandemic. WHO, likely cowed by China, was loath to acknowledge any information or to accept any help from Taiwan. As we mentioned in chapter 1, WHO official Bruce Aylward provided some rare comic relief during the crisis. He stonewalled and then hung up during an interview with a Hong Kong-based news source when he was asked whether WHO would reconsider Taiwan's membership request. The same news source had reported in February that Aylward, "who has decades of experience in battling disease outbreaks, led a WHO mission to Wuhan, several weeks after the pandemic started. After returning, he told the media the country had 'absolutely turned it around.'" Further, "In a clip shared by Chinese media, Aylward said the country knew what it was doing and 'if I had COVID-19 I'd want to be treated in China,' he said."

Taiwan's health minister Chen Shih-chung wrote a letter to WHO at the end of December 2019, warning that the new virus could be transmitted from person to person.[14] According to the same report, "WHO, in a statement to Reuters, said they didn't receive an email about person-to-person transmission." The article also reminded readers, "As late as Jan. 14, the WHO said 'there was no evidence of human-to-human transmission' of the virus." WHO declared the outbreak a pandemic in March.

After the Aylward incident and other similar snubs, Taiwan's officials and press responded by ramping up their criticism of WHO. They accused the UN of botching the response and showing too much deference to Beijing. WHO's director general, Tedros Adhanom Ghebreyesus, said this criticism was—this will not come as a shock to American readers—"racist."[15] Tedros may have been stinging from a petition originating in Taiwan asking for his ouster.[16] Even through late April, he was still officially denying that Taiwan warned WHO about human-to-human transmission.[17]

In the future, Taiwan may ask the United States or Singapore to notify WHO officials. Information from non-Taiwanese sources might be easier to stomach. Assuming, of course, the United States is still funding WHO.

SWEDEN

Everybody wants to talk about Sweden, maybe because they can't find Taiwan on a map. Or they can't remember Belgium or the UK, both of which had higher death rates than Sweden. So did Andorra, Spain, Italy, and France. All worse than Sweden. All locked down. True, Norway next door, with half Sweden's population, had a lower death rate. But so did Japan, which never locked down.

Famously, the Swedish government decided to follow the commonsense suggestions of Anders Tegnell, an epidemiologist at Sweden's independent Public Health Agency. He advised voluntary "trust-based" measures, such as washing your hands and staying away from sick people.

"This is not a disease that can be stopped or eradicated," he told *Nature* magazine in April, "at least until a working vaccine is produced."[18] As a result, he surmised, there's no point in trying to absolutely stop or eradicate it. The Swedish government was vindicated for following this advice, since, as we have shown, there's no clear evidence that lockdowns elsewhere did much good—and plenty of evidence that they did harm.

It was a close call, though. Sweden, like the UK and United States, has its fill of experts. When they heard the government was going to heed Tegnell's advice, 22 "high-profile" scientists wrote an open letter urging lockdowns.[19] In late March, another petition "signed by more than 2,000 doctors, scientists, and professors" asked the government to reverse course.[20] Again, "high-profile" people think it's their birthright to impose their wisdom on the masses. Trust us—we're gods.

It was clear by the end of April that the calm and reasonable approach was working. The gods were wrong. In an interview with the BBC on April 24, Tegnell noted that, as he had expected, "almost half the fatalities have come from nursing homes."[21] The same trend was observed in many places with lockdowns.[22] In a rare display of humble leadership, Tegnell said in May that he might change his mind if the data proved his strategy wasn't working.[23]

On social media, though, it looked like many wanted Sweden's strategy to fail. Folks kept digging into the data to find proof that Sweden had really done worse than reported. The main tactic was simple confirmation bias: mention only those countries that had lockdowns and lower death rates. What about countries with lockdowns and worse rates? Those didn't count because they were too far away from Sweden. Like Belgium.

For example, in mid-May a computer scientist claimed that "Sweden has now the highest #covid19 fatality rate per million population of the world. A direct consequence of the inhumane 'herd immunity' plan."[24] He then showed a plot of *daily* per capita death rate, where on May 15 Sweden did indeed fare worse per capita than the UK and Belgium. (Sweden had 117 reported coronavirus deaths that day, or 11.5 per million. The UK reported 384, or 6.9 per million, and Belgium reported 56, or 4.9 per million.) Some in the press used this same trick around the same time. The *Telegraph* reported, "Sweden becomes country with highest coronavirus death rate per capita." They said, "Sweden had 6.08 deaths per million inhabitants per day on a rolling seven-day average between May 13 and May 20. This is the highest in the world...."[25]

It's a trick because once the deaths fall to near zero it's easy for any random country to come out on top of the death toll for any given day, especially if they have small populations. And at that time deaths were plummeting for every country in Europe. Suppose, for example, that it's the last day of the pandemic. Nobody dies from the bug in the UK or Belgium, or anywhere else, but one person dies in Sweden. Headlines could trumpet, "Sweden worst in the world!" Comparing individual days is absurd, but it happened. All to gin up fear.

Less than a month before, around April 18, at the height of the pandemic in Europe, there had been a huge spike in death rates—in Belgium, to about four times higher than Sweden's at the time. Overall, Belgium, with 10 percent more people than Sweden, had more than twice as many per capita deaths. Yet no one, and especially not this computer scientist, said that was a direct result of Belgium's lockdown.

It was popular to compare Sweden to Norway during the crisis, because Norway is close to Sweden and had even fewer deaths per capita. But Norway's population, only half as large as Sweden's, is far more spread out. Moreover, in late May Camille Stoltenberg, the head of the Norwegian Institute of Public Health, admitted: "Our assessment now...is that we could possibly have achieved the same effects and avoided some of the unfortunate impacts by not locking down, but by instead keeping open but with infection control measures."[26]

JAPAN

The default thinking of most respectable people was that lockdowns work and must be mandatory. A representative headline from March 14 from *Foreign Policy* magazine said, "Japan's Halfhearted Coronavirus Measures Are Working Anyway: Despite Indifferent Lockdowns and

Poor Testing, Japan Seems to Be Skipping the Worst of the Pandemic."[27] The article said, "In its battle with the coronavirus Japan appears to be doing everything wrong."

Here's a better way to put this: in its reporting on Japan's coronavirus strategy, *Foreign Policy* did everything wrong.

Japan, population 127 million, had a death rate of about 7 per million. This is 73 times *lower* than the UK's roughly 511 per million as of May 18. If Japan was doing it wrong, wrong was the right way to go. All countries should have been following Japan, which didn't lock down. On May 25, Prime Minister Shinzo Abe announced the end of Japan's state of emergency. The country attributed 851 deaths to coronavirus, or 6.7 per 100,000. That was one of the lowest rates of any developed country.[28]

Throughout the non-lockdown, journalists couldn't stop hectoring Japan. In April, the BBC claimed, "Coronavirus: Japan's low testing rate raises questions."[29] The *New Statesman* entitled its piece, "How Japan's Refusal to Impose a Coronavirus Lockdown is Dividing the Country."[30] They didn't mention that it might also be saving lives. Some predicted that Japan was sure to get it in the neck.[31] The idea that lockdowns might not work seemed unthinkable.

Japan's strategy was much like Taiwan's. The government restricted flights and delayed school openings. On subways, the Japanese wore masks, which is common anyway, and so on. The response to the virus in Japan was so relaxed that one report said, "COVID-19 did not change much in Japan's daily life."[32] Indeed, some credited the laid-back attitude for a 20 percent drop in suicides.[33] "People spending more time at home with their families," the *Guardian* reported, "fewer people were commuting to work and delays to the start of the school year are seen as factors in the fall." By May, even *Science* magazine was reporting how Japan had fought the coronavirus without nuking its economy. The country, it said, "drove down the number of daily new cases to near target levels of 0.5 per 100,000 people with voluntary and not very restrictive social distancing and without large-scale testing...."[34]

Who knows what drove the numbers down? We don't have two Japans to compare. Or two Swedens, or two Taiwans. What we do know is that these places chose not to tank their economies the way so many other countries did, and the coronavirus doesn't seem to have punished them for that as much as the press has.

SOUTH KOREA AND MORE

South Korea had a death rate of about 5 per million. The South Koreans didn't lock down, but they did aggressively track people with the disease. Hong Kong didn't have a lockdown either and it had about 0.5 deaths per million. These countries didn't sit on their hands. They just didn't join the planetary panic. Nor did they suffer as many predicted they would.

In the U.S., 8 states never locked down.[35] They were, with deaths per million in late June: Iowa (111), Oklahoma (73), Nebraska (64), North Dakota (56), South Dakota (50), Arkansas (32), Utah (25), and Wyoming (14).[36] Wyoming has about 580 thousand people, and had only 8 coronavirus deaths.

The states with the harshest lockdowns were California (83 deaths per million), Illinois (330), Michigan (490), New York (1,162), and New Jersey (1,166).

Now there are many more differences between states besides lockdown status. But using these comparisons, there's no way to claim the lockdowns succeeded. Almost all of California's deaths were in the Los Angeles area; most in Illinois were in or around Chicago; Michigan's were around Detroit; and New York and New Jersey's were in the New York City metropolitan area. So population density surely played a role. Yet these entire states had to endure lockdowns, even places far from the population centers.

Many experts and journalists were so sure we needed lockdowns that they predicted disaster for states that opened up. Learning nothing from recent events, the *New York Times* trotted out "models" that "project[ed] sharp rise in deaths as states reopen."[37] Anthony Fauci wrung his hands and warned that the "consequences could be really serious" if states opened "prematurely."[38]

The most hysterical forecasts were about Georgia, one of the first states to open up—on April 30.[39] The experts and pundits were sure that mass death would follow as surely night follows day. The *Washington Post* ran a piece under the headline: "Georgia Leads the Race to Become America's No. 1 Death Destination."[40] Classy, but wrong. When that didn't happen, some of the press took to reporting not new deaths, but total deaths tied to the coronavirus.[41] Of course, total deaths can only go up—they are still going up even as rates drop to zero. A model that CNN touted at the end of April said deaths in the state could double![42] Sadly for the doomsayers, Georgia's death rate kept falling.[43]

The experts and their media megaphones were so sure they were right that they would not, or could not, see the data that proved them wrong.

CHAPTER 14

LESSONS LEARNED

The trick to forgetting the big picture is to look at everything close up.

—*Chuck Palahniuk*[1]

Baby Boomers recall stories from parents and grandparents about the last World War and the Great Depression that came before it. They were dystopian tales of hardship and fear and suffering that seemed unreal to us when we heard them in much better times. We call the people who endured those years the Greatest Generation.

Maybe our current trials don't compare. Still, these days are surely the most unsettling ones we've seen. When we make it through, will we have learned anything? Will we have wisdom to pass down to younger generations?

We're still too close to some of these things, such as the violent riots that broke out around the country in late May of 2020. Deep reflection takes time and distance that we don't yet have.

But we have lived through weeks and months of the coronavirus crisis. We know enough to draw some conclusions. And we should. The world economy and our basic rights and health are still under assault. Even with deaths dropping in the summer, a rise in "cases" scared some state officials into locking down again. If and when a "second wave" hits in the fall or winter, there will be immense pressure to replay the 2020 playbook. And even if that doesn't happen, there's always the next pandemic. Perhaps worst of all, we're being told that we can never go back to the way we lived before; instead, we'll just have to get used to "the new normal."

LOCAL OVER GLOBAL

We can't undo the technology that connects us to all the world all the time. But we've seen firsthand the problems that come from living in that technology. In the future, we should hold ourselves to a healthier standard. Through most of history, people noticed truly huge calamities only when they forced themselves upon their attention. Londoners needed no press campaign to shelter in Underground stations in 1940 when the sound of buzz bombs and the Luftwaffe echoed through the streets. Those sounds spoke for themselves. Zero dissent. Everyone was on the same page.

Eighty years later, we have both gained and lost something. We weren't made to be everywhere at once. We were made to be where we are. If we want to benefit from knowing in real time what is happening around the world—without giving undue weight to events that are hard to judge at a distance—we need to make it a higher priority to be present locally. When social and traditional media are calling for panic, balance that message with what you see when you unplug and take a walk. Throughout the crisis, we all knew local facts that contradicted the panic porn bombarding our eyes and ears. Perhaps you were surprised to see a death certificate that listed COVID-19 as the cause of death. Or maybe a healthy fifty-something friend tested positive but had a mild case, or no symptoms at all. Or you heard about empty hospital wards and laid-off nurses, and yet couldn't schedule a cancer screening.

And still you, or someone you know, discounted the direct evidence of eyes and ears in favor of a digital simulacrum.

If we had all focused on what we knew, up close and personal, things might have unfolded differently. If the experts scream that the sky is falling, and yet it stays put when you take your walk, then you might not want to treat their advice as gospel.

BALANCE EXPERT ADVICE WITH COMMON SENSE

But often, expert warnings are not so easy to judge. Their reasons for ginning up a panic will seem credible at first. In that case, step back, take a deep breath, and recall a few key points.

First of all, it's the experts' duty to convince you, the citizen, in plain English, of what they fear and what they want you to do about it. Maybe their dire warnings sound credible dressed up in technical language. But we must still insist that they explain it in a way that will allow us to judge its wisdom. We must demand that if we want to keep government by the people, rather than by the experts.

The fact is, we almost always have more time than they are telling us. And in most cases the panicked response is not going to be the ideal response. If a credible authority calls for prompt, reasonable action, by all means get on board. But don't be stampeded into imprudent choices. And if, in hindsight, the call was wrong, demand a change in course.

Over the last several months, we have learned a lot. We just had a costly course on preventative hygiene, for example. We didn't ask for it, but let's not let it go to waste. The sensible low-cost measures—such as more hand washing—become good habits that can reduce the spread of future infections. Many things that we can do freely for ourselves make sense, even if they don't scale up to a national pandemic-stopper.

TAKE CARE OF THE MOST VULNERABLE

From the beginning, we should have focused our efforts on the most vulnerable, namely, the sick and elderly. Instead, in some places we did the opposite. To free up hospital beds, some states "ordered nursing homes to accept patients with active COVID-19 infections who were being discharged from hospitals."[2] Really. What's shameful is that they kept at it, even when it had become clear that the projected numbers for needed hospital beds was way too high. On April 23, Governor Andrew Cuomo of New York was still saying that nursing homes had "no right to object" to these patients.[3]

Health care expert Betsy McCaughey described the tragedy this way: "The carnage started in March, when hospitals inundated with COVID-19 patients insisted on clearing out elderly patients, even if they were still infected, and sending them to whatever nursing homes had empty beds. To swing that, they had to get rid of a safety regulation requiring patients to test negative twice for COVID-19 before being placed in a home. The state Health Department willingly complied."[4]

Meanwhile, the USNS *Comfort* and the Javits Center in New York sat unoccupied, with thousands of empty hospital beds.

In part due to these mistakes, about 42 percent of recorded COVID-19 deaths in the United States were in nursing homes or residential care facilities.[5]

Florida governor Ron DeSantis took the right approach. He studied early evidence from other countries, such as South Korea and Italy, and noticed the much greater risk for the elderly. As a result, he focused on protecting retirement communities and nursing homes. On March 15, DeSantis issued an executive order prohibiting visits to nursing homes and preventing sick patients from being transferred to them.[6] At the same time, he shored up hospital resources[7] and gave counties space to tailor their responses to local conditions.[8]

Those are all steps that we should take in the future.

TAKE MODELS AND PREDICTIONS WITH A PINCH OF SALT

Predicting the weather is child's play compared to predicting what billions of people will do during an event unlike anything we have ever seen before. If we had applied the skepticism with which we view the fourteen-day weather forecast to the Imperial College model, things would have been different. The coronavirus would have done what it did. But we could have avoided the bigger mess.

To his credit, New York governor Andrew Cuomo learned to carry a saltshaker with him. In late May, some parts of New York state started to reopen, but not the Big Apple. He refused to predict when the hardest-hit American city would open, but he also (wisely) refused to let expert predictions dictate. "Now, people can speculate, people can guess, I think next week, I think two weeks, I think a month," he said. "I'm out of that business, because we all failed at that business. All the early national experts, here's my projection, here's my projection model, they were all wrong, they were all wrong."[9]

BEWARE THE OVERCONFIDENCE OF EXPERTS

Expert advice is like bright light—useful when pointed in the right direction but blinding otherwise. The coronavirus pandemic offers both leaders and citizens three lessons on how to make the best use of such advice.

First, experts are often wrong—especially about the future.[10] We saw this in two ways as the coronavirus crisis played out. One was that experts made bad predictions. The Imperial College model was certainly a prime example, but there were dozens of others. Politicians, the press, and the public swallowed many claims just because they came from official sources.

Another was contradictory claims. Whether it was masks or surface cleaning or death rates, different experts kept saying different things, and in some cases the same experts said different things.

The second lesson is that most experts don't get the first lesson. They see how it applies to other experts, but they rarely apply it to themselves. Prior to the panic, authorities such as WHO could be quite candid about what they didn't know. But when widespread panic set in and everyone expected experts to render prompt and precise answers, they seemed to have a hard time admitting, *We don't know.*

Next time, instead of expecting them to admit that, just assume it.

The third lesson is that knowledge is not the same thing as wisdom. Most experts work in silos.[11] Their shared confidence in their expertise often leaks, causing them to be cocksure even when they've wandered outside their domain of knowledge.

This is an acute problem when experts are advising on a massively complex problem like a pandemic. No mere mortal knew everything about the new coronavirus, or everything that would have been good to know, especially when the virus was first spreading. Think of all the relevant domains: virology, epidemiology, statistics, internal medicine, emergency medicine, nursing, pathology, pharmacology, physiology, molecular biology, geriatrics, social psychology, global economics, public policy, constitutional law, international law, law enforcement, communications, journalism, technology, small business, big business, education, child protection, social services, transportation and logistics, and more.

No one can master all of that. So we can only solve such complex problems with input from a wide variety of experts. It falls to our elected leaders to weigh their advice, mustering whatever wisdom and prudence they can.[12]

This may have been our single largest mistake in the coronavirus episode: one narrow, untested analysis got a viral boost before all relevant wisdom could be heard. And then politicians, once committed to that analysis, found it hard to pivot in the face of new and contrary evidence.

Experts have their place, but sometimes they need to be put in their place.

Choose Freedom over Central Planning

In the last century, the great Austrian economist F. A. Hayek showed why no government can plan an economy. Only someone with omniscience could know all that would need to be known for this.[13] Mere mortals don't stand a chance.

Governments tend to produce one-size-fits-nobody plans that presume that the same thing is true for all people in all situations. But individuals know much more about their own needs than bureaucrats do.

Americans were spared some of the worst excesses of central control during the pandemic. But the United States could have opted for far more local freedom and discernment. In fact, most people were changing their behavior before the lockdowns. One report (worryingly, based on cell phone records) said that in the six states tracked, "23 percent of people were staying home on average during the first week of March" *before* lockdown orders were issued. This "proportion jumped to 47 percent a month later."[14]

Nothing that the three of us have seen makes us think this did much to slow the spread of the virus, but that's not the point. The point is that well-informed free people do about as well as people under compulsion—and with far less collateral damage.

TAKE TRADITIONAL MEDIA CAUTIOUSLY

On May 24, 2020—Sunday of Memorial Day weekend—the *New York Times* went for drama. Rather than the usual mix of stories and pictures on its front page, the Grey Lady printed a thousand names from the tens of thousands of deaths tied to COVID-19. The headline read, paradoxically, "US Deaths Near 100,000, an Incalculable Loss." The list also scrolled on the main page of the paper's website, like a dynamic Vietnam War memorial.[15]

In almost any other context, a list of casualties like this would have been touching. Yet we couldn't help but see it as part of a tiresome effort to keep the fear going. Americans in droves had started ignoring guidelines in states still under lockdown, from California to Maryland. And they kept on doing so, despite this effort on the part of America's paper of record.

The *Times* proudly posted an image of the cover on Twitter on Saturday night. The Drudge Report, still in full-tilt panic mode, posted it at the top of its page. Dozens of spin-off articles reported on the cover—stories about a story—in another media exercise in self-reference.

Before it went to print, though, the paper had to correct the story. The *sixth* name on the list, twenty-seven-year-old Jordan Driver Haynes, had been a rare death under thirty. But he did not die of COVID-19. He was murdered.[16]

Even in the pandemic panic, there were a few points of light and good sense in the mainstream press—if you knew where to look. Joe Nocera expressed doubts about the wisdom of the lockdowns at Bloomberg.[17] Nate Silver, a rare journalist who is also an expert statistician, often corrected media mistakes. The *Wall Street Journal* editorial page even hosted a debate.

Still, the incentives of the mainstream press push them to stoke fear—especially if such fear may harm a hated politician or despised cause. If you forget this one-way force when you consume media, you will be a slave to every headline and every update. And you will become part of a great collective force that can spur elected officials to make bad calls just so the public can see them doing something. If you don't want to join that force, then you must steel yourself against the press's constant stoking of panic.

With enough public resistance, the mainstream press might even rethink its conduct. Those of us who remember when the morning paper could scoop the evening news and vice versa shake our heads. How times have changed. Too bad the *Times* hasn't changed with them. Forty-five percent of the world's people now use smartphones, so mainline media aren't going to scoop anyone anymore. They can't compete with 3.5 billion independent reporters, so maybe it's time they stopped trying.

But they could do something to win back some of their erstwhile respect. Instead of keeping up the futile competition with social media, why don't they become what social media can't be? They can't break the story first, but they could strive to give the most honest, reasoned, balanced take on it.

And as for the rest of us, why not expect more from our news sources?

Even if that's a hopeless cause, we don't have to be carried along by the press's fear mongering, which can change from week to week. At first, the scare story was that American hospitals were going to be overwhelmed, as in Italy with its subpar socialized medicine.[18] Then, when people could see that the hospitals weren't overrun—in fact, many of them were mostly empty—we were going to run out of ventilators.[19] When that didn't happen, patients and healthcare workers were going to die for lack of masks and other PPE.[20] When that failed to occur, the new disaster was a shortage of tests.[21] Instead, soon, testing centers were closing because supply outstripped demand.[22] The press then told us that President Trump was going to cut testing to hide the second wave of deaths that would follow the reckless easing up on the lockdowns.[23]

To fortify ourselves against this week's new panic, we may just need to cast our minds back to last week's scare story.

MAKE SOCIAL MEDIA ACCOUNTABLE

Content on social media stirred panic over the coronavirus. But so did the platforms themselves. Facebook and YouTube validated official opinion and censored unapproved opinion even from genuine experts. Rather than providing open platforms for debate, they've become creepy protectors of the party line.

How do we stop this from happening again? We're highly skeptical of calls to make these platforms public utilities. What would probably happen in that case is what economists call "regulatory capture." Instead of having private companies policing speech, as we have now, we'd have public-private mongrels doing the same, only with more power.

There is one strategy, though, that could help. Facebook, Twitter, and other such companies enjoy the legal status of neutral platforms. In this way, they're like AT&T and Verizon. They're not responsible for third-party content, so they can't be punished because a third party commits libel on their platform.

That would be fair if they really were neutral—if they treated posts and tweets the way Verizon and AT&T treat phone calls. But they're not, as we have seen over and over again. Right now, they get to have their cake and eat it too. All because of the 1996 Communications Decency Act, which mandates that "no provider or user of an interactive computer service shall be treated as the publisher or speaker of any information provided by another information content provider."

These firms should have to choose: either act like neutral platforms and allow anyone to post any content that's legal or lose the legal privilege of being treated like one. In the latter case, they would be treated as publishers, legally liable for everything that's posted on their platforms.

We're pretty sure they'd prefer the advantage of neutrality.

Loyal Opposition

Our final suggestion is only a germ of an idea. In British government, the loyal opposition refers to the party that opposes the governing party while remaining loyal to the Crown. If you've ever watched parliamentary proceedings, you know the debate there is at least as acrimonious as in the U.S. Congress. But the concept is gold—a body of people committed both to critiquing the dominant voice in leadership and to the common good.

In the present case, the dominant voice isn't a political party, but rather official experts. But if a small group, whether politicians or vetted scientists, has vast power to control the rest of us, then others must have power to contest them. The coronavirus panic and shutdown would not have played out as it did if a few scientific experts, boosted by a reckless media, had not had so much unchecked power.

Elected representatives need to be able to weigh competing advice. But the dominant point of view tends to marginalize all dissent. This is what we saw over and over during the pandemic.

Perhaps an official loyal opposition could temper this all-too-human tendency. Its sole job would be to probe, question, and where warranted, dismantle the official advice our political leaders receive. Of course, the experts in this opposing role would also be fallible. Still, the cut and thrust between the two sides might reveal some otherwise hidden truths.

We don't know whether our suggestions here would have prevented the catastrophe in 2020. But we do know this: we must do something to check the power of official experts over our lives.

AGAINST THE BRAVE NEW NORMAL

Of all tyrannies, a tyranny sincerely exercised for the good of its victim may be the most oppressive. It may be better to live under robber barons than under omnipotent moral busybodies. The robber baron's cruelty may sometimes sleep, his cupidity may at some point be satiated, but those who torment us for our own good will torment us without end, for they do so with the approval of their conscience.

—C. S. Lewis[1]

When modern Americans think of tyranny, we picture dictators of the recent past: Stalin, Hitler, Mao, Mussolini. When the American Founders thought of tyranny, they pictured kings, and parliaments, and mobs. They knew from their study of history to fear the tyranny of the majority.

We got a taste of this in 2020. In their panic, most Americans supported the lockdowns. We were inspired not by mere deference to authority, but by fear and a concern for others. Cities, states, and the federal government overstepped their bounds. And it wasn't okay just because most people agreed to it. That's why our basic rights—to assemble, to the exercise our religion freely, and so forth—are enshrined in the Constitution. That guarantee is crucial because the government, riding some rising wave of public opinion, will always be tempted to disregard the rights of even a balky and resistant minority.

It must have been fear, and the hatred it can spawn, that led at least one person to turn arsonist. The First Pentecostal Church in Holly

Springs, Mississippi, had held services in compliance with state restrictions, which classified churches as essential businesses. Cities were free to impose stricter measures, but not to change that classification. When the city interrupted services, the church sued.

Someone was so incensed that the church challenged local orders that he torched the building and spray painted "BET YOU STAY HOME NOW YOU HYPOKRITS" in the parking lot.[2] We presume the arsonist judged the city to be in the right. But then, their version of justice calls their judgment into question. Whatever you make of the church's decision to sue, it wasn't hypocrisy. They, not the arsonist, were squarely within the American tradition.

Petty Tyrants

According to one report, Michigan governor Gretchen Whitmer said her orders to state residents "have the force of law, so they are 'not suggestions, not optional or helpful hints.'"[3] Never mind that her orders were not duly enacted laws. Also, she seemed to think that the rules were not for me, but for thee. After she had told citizens to avoid "inessential" trips to recreate on Michigan's lakes, it came out that her husband had asked the dock service at the Whitmers' lake house to put their boat in the water for Memorial Day weekend.[4] She also tried to use the crisis to funnel taxpayer money to a Democrat group for contact tracing, denied she had done so, was called out on that, and then blew off the accusations. But the public scrutiny forced her to cancel the contract.[5] The money would have gone to "EveryAction, a firm that is closely linked to NGP VAN, a technology provider that boasts that it powers 'nearly every major Democratic campaign in America.'"[6]

Whitmer was not the only one to grab for power in the crisis. Besides goading citizens to rat each other out, New York City mayor Bill de Blasio became livid when groups of Orthodox Jews were still holding funerals during his lockdown. He thundered that his "message to the Jewish community, and all communities, is this simple: the time for warnings has passed."[7] De Blasio's focus on Jewish funerals raised suspicions that anti-Semitism might be at play. Those suspicions seemed to be confirmed when city officials welded shut the entrance to a playground in a Jewish neighborhood while tolerating mass gatherings of left-wing protesters.[8] Strangely, politicians' heavy-handed enforcement of the lockdown seemed to evaporate when protests-turned-riots erupted in late May following the horrific death of George Floyd at the hands of Minneapolis cop Derek Chauvin. We can't prove but we do suspect that the unprecedented joblessness and despair caused by the lockdowns fed the rioting, as some have suggested.[9]

We also know that the protests and riots exposed the naked hypocrisy of the press, politicians, and public health officials. They exempted and even encouraged protesters and rioters while scolding everyone else. On June 5, over a thousand health professionals wrote an open letter defending mass protests for the sake of…public health. "We believe that the way forward is not to suppress protests in the name of public health," they argued, "but to respond to protesters demands in the name of public health, thereby addressing multiple public health crises."

And, for the most part, the press played along. On June 13, *Time* tweeted two headlines only a half hour apart. The first approvingly heralded the "physicians'" letter mentioned above.[10] The second headline read glumly, "Hundreds of Far-Right Protesters Defy COVID-19 Restrictions to Demonstrate in London."[11]

The next day, NBC News ran the following two headlines a little more than an hour apart: "Rally for Black Trans Lives Draws Packed Crowd to Brooklyn Museum Plaza," and "President Trump Plans to Rally His Supporters Next Saturday for the First Time Since Most of the Country Was Shuttered by the Coronavirus. But Health Experts Are Questioning That Decision."[12] On June 22, *Newsweek* matched that feat with these back-to-back stories: "'No Evidence' Black Lives Matter Protests Causes COVID-19 Spike: Study," and "Oklahoma Reports Highest Ever Daily COVID-19 Cases after Trump Tulsa Rally."[13] We could go on and on about the riots and pride parades and anti-cop zones that got a pass in the press while the plebes were still expected to huddle at home. But no doubt you witnessed all this firsthand. After this spectacle, why would anyone still trust the press, politicians, and public health officials on the risks of COVID-19? We wrote this book in part to expose their bad faith. We hardly expected them to display it with such reckless abandon.

NEVER LET A CRISIS GO TO WASTE

From the start of the crisis, some in Washington smelled a chance to expand government power. Just as the Senate was finishing bipartisan negotiations on its first coronavirus relief bill, House Speaker Nancy Pelosi managed to kill it. Suddenly the Democrats wanted to lard any bill with their pet projects, from abortion funding and restriction of carbon emissions on airlines to mandatory minimum wages on any businesses receiving help. Echoing Rahm Emmanuel, South Carolina representative James Clyburn told the Democratic caucus that the bill was "a tremendous opportunity to restructure things to fit our vision."[14] After their first effort failed, House Democrats tried again in mid-May with the $3 trillion HEROES Act. It offered $1,200 to each illegal immigrant and a million dollars to the National Science Foundation to study "misinformation" related to the coronavirus.[15] On April 2, California governor Gavin Newsom admitted that the pandemic was an "opportunity" to pursue a new, progressive agenda. The cover theme of the April 20–27 issue of *The Nation* was "How Not to Waste This Crisis." And the UN Climate Change Fund called it an "opportunity to change the world."

All these folks were following a well-thumbed playbook. As Robert Higgs shows in *Crisis and Leviathan*, national crises have been the progressive tool of choice for government expansion. For that purpose, the 2020 pandemic panic worked better and faster than any previous crisis, and with nary a shot fired. Progressives have often spoken wistfully of "the moral equivalent of war," a shared peacetime goal that inspires sacrificial devotion.[16] The coronavirus pandemic provided just that. If millions of deaths were the alternative, short-term lockdowns and even martial law might make sense. But the only reason to think that millions could die was predictive models that were just fancy guesses—bad ones, as it turned out.

Donald Trump had better instincts. Trump had tweeted in March that the cure should not be worse than the disease. The hostile response was deafening. Did people want a worse cure? No. But the officially smart people were predicting a historic catastrophe, and who was he to raise questions? In the end, most state and national governments acted accordingly—not just here, but around the world.

"Science" told them to. After a judge struck down her executive order against religious groups, the governor of Oregon explained, "The science behind these executive orders hasn't changed one bit."[17] In early March, Democratic presidential nominee Joe Biden, who just weeks earlier had lambasted President Trump for restricting travel from China, said that his campaign would "lead by science." The lockdowns, "social distancing," and mask mandates were imposed hastily, without public debate. "In a matter of weeks," noted the *New York Times*, "millions of Americans have been asked to do what would have been unthinkable only a few months ago: Don't go to work, don't go to school, don't leave the house at all, unless you have to."[18] Now clever people are telling us to treat our cramped life under these outlandish restraints as "the new normal." We wrote this book to defend the normal normal. Americans have become too fearful, too fragile. But as we have seen, that's just part of the story. The other part is that fallible experts have gained far too much power over the commanding heights of culture. Even when they meant well, they didn't know what they pretended to know. Worse, they used the pretense of knowledge to turn not just our fears, but also our good intentions against us.

A WAY FORWARD

Which way will we go? We don't want to become East Germany, or even Western Europe. Consider the European Commission's Roadmap on Vaccination document, prepared in March 2019, a year before the crisis. It recommended that EU citizens be forced to carry their vaccination status on their passports.[19] The years 2019–2021 were to be used for a "Feasibility study for the development of a common EU vaccination card." The "common vaccination card/passport for EU citizens" would arrive in 2022. Nor do we want to follow the one-worlders at the World Economic Forum, who pounced on the pandemic as a chance to launch their creepy "great reset." What's that? It is, as they explain,

- A commitment to jointly and urgently build the foundations of our economic and social system for a more fair, sustainable and resilient future
- A new social contract centred on human dignity, social justice and where societal progress does not fall behind economic development
- The global health crisis has laid bare longstanding ruptures in our economies and societies, and created a social crisis that urgently requires decent, meaningful jobs[20]

Yeah, right. No one should be surprised that globalist technocrats, just having witnessed a grand social experiment, are now licking their chops. Making people carry papers to prove their immunity?[21] One-world semi-socialism? These started as conspiracy theories, not suggestions. And we're pretty sure that neither is quite fit for American tastes.

A more likely road to serfdom in the United States could be paved by big tech. In late March, some techno-utopians were already sketching out the solution to the pandemic. In *Wired* magazine, Tristan Harris called for digital platforms to provide their billions of users with a "corrective lens" to help them conform their beliefs and behavior more quickly to the new reality. "This emergency, this moment," he wrote, "calls for a fundamentally new approach to technology—to abandon the myth of neutral metrics and engagement, and restructure technology to prioritize this corrective lens that can help save millions of lives."[22] Despotism, if it arrives on our shores, may not come wearing a swastika or hammer and sickle, or even a blue helmet. It could come bearing promises of safety, enlightenment, and stock options.

But there's a countervailing spirit in our country. Even early on, there were hopeful signs that we had not wholly succumbed to fear. When New York mayor Bill de Blasio set up an e-hotline for residents to rat out their neighbors by sending in pictures of offenders, it was flooded with pictures of, well, manhood, Hitler memes, and extended middle fingers.[23] And on Independence Day 2020, when petty tyrants such as California governor Gavin Newsom and Los Angeles mayor Eric Garcetti banned fireworks displays, L.A. residents responded by lighting up the skies.[24]

This defiance, earthy and small as it is, gives us hope that our country won't embrace the Brave New Normal. If we don't learn the right lessons from the 2020 pandemic panic, though, it could sneak up, settle in, and cost us our lives, our fortunes, and our sacred honor.

Acknowledgments

We never could have written this book under such a tight deadline without the help of friends and family. Our many thanks to Ginny Richards for reading and commenting on the manuscript and for formatting all the notes. Thanks also to Robert Čihák, Jonathan Witt, Don Galbadage, and Anita Axe for their careful reading and comments on a near-complete manuscript.

Thanks finally to Tom Spence and Elizabeth Kantor at Regnery, without whom this book never could have happened, and to Gillian Richards, our copyeditor at Regnery, who caught many glitches, typos, and infelicities.

We bear responsibility for any mistakes remaining.

Notes

Introduction

1. Thomas Sowell, "Random Thoughts on the Passing Scene," *Capitalism Magazine*, September 22, 2005, https://www.capitalismmagazine.com/2005/09/random-thoughts-september-2005.
2. Jeffrey Cook, Clayton Sandell, and Jennifer Leong, "Former Police Officer Arrested in Park for Throwing Ball with Daughter Due to Coronavirus Social Distancing Rules," ABC News, April 8, 2020, https://abcnews.go.com/US/police-officer-arrested-park-throwing-ball-daughter-due/story?id=70032966.
3. Renatta Signorini, "State Police Cite PA Woman for 'Going for a Drive' amid Stay-at-Home Order," *Pittsburgh Tribune-Review*, April 3, 2020, https://triblive.com/news/pennsylvania/state-troopers-cite-pa-woman-for-going-for-a-drive-amid-stay-at-home-order.
4. Giulia McDonnell Nieto del Rio and Theresa Waldrop, "99-Year-Old in New Jersey Charged after Attending Party during State Ban on Gatherings," CNN, April 2, 2020, https://www.cnn.com/2020/04/02/us/99-year-old-charged-new-jersey-coronavirus/index.html.
5. "New Jersey COVID-19 Information Hub," Official Site of the State of New Jersey, accessed July 28, 2020, https://covid19.nj.gov/forms/violation.
6. "'Snitches Get Rewards': Garcetti Issues New Rules for Construction Sites, Encourages Community to Report Safer at Home Violators,"

CBS Los Angeles, March 31, 2020, https://losangeles.cbslocal.com/2020/03/31/coronavirus-los-angeles-eric-garcetti-snitches-get-rewards.

7. Muriel Bowser (@MayorBowser), "2/ After a long meeting, it expressed its frustration about people not staying home, and consequently, that its stops may be delayed this year. We agreed that road closures will be necessary for the Easter Bunny to quickly hop its way through the District and stay on time," Twitter, April 12, 2020, 9:41 a.m., https://twitter.com/MayorBowser/status/1249331835873693698.

8. Christina Capatides, "'Shoot Them Dead': Philippine President Rodrigo Duterte Orders Police and Military to Kill Citizens Who Defy Coronavirus Lockdown," CBS News, April 2, 2020, https://www.cbsnews.com/amp/news/rodrigo-duterte-philippines-president-coronavirus-lockdown-shoot-people-dead.

9. President Trump, "Remarks by President Trump, Vice President Pence, and Members of the Coronavirus Task Force in Press Briefing," April 8, 2020, https://www.whitehouse.gov/briefings-statements/remarks-president-trump-vice-president-pence-members-coronavirus-task-force-press-briefing-22.

10. "COVID-19 Projections," Institute for Health Metrics & Evaluation, https://covid19.healthdata.org/united-states-of-america; Andrew C. McCarthy, "COVID-19 Projection Models Are Proving to Be Unreliable," *National Review*, April 9, 2020, https://www.nationalreview.com/corner/coronavirus-pandemic-projection-models-proving-unreliable.

11. Fox News, "Dr. Fauci on Criticism of Coronavirus Modeling," YouTube, April 10, 2020, https://www.youtube.com/watch?v=URZB0Cp0mW0.

12. Jacob Knutson, "Fauci Says Trump Backed Off Easter Reopening after Seeing Coronavirus Projections," Axios, March 30, 2020, https://www.axios.com/coronavirus-fauci-trump-easter-reopening-deaths-210eeeac-7281-41da-9a5f-935679fe1ee3.html.

13. Institute for Health Metrics and Evaluation (@IHME_UW), "We strongly agree that decision-makers shoud draw on a diversity of COVID-19 models. We're committed to scientific debate and constant improvement of our predictions. Learn more, http://healthdata.org/covid/faqs," April 11, 2020, 7:00 a.m., https://twitter.com/IHME_UW/status/1248928788353875970.

14. Umair Irfan, "2 New Studies Show Shutdowns Were Astonishingly Effective," Vox, June 9, 2020, https://www.vox.com/2020/6/9/21284087/coronavirus-covid-19-shutdown-lockdown-cases-deaths?__c=1.

15. By April 13, the public's patience with the mandated shutdowns was growing thin. Still, an Ipsos poll showed that most Americans were still worried about the virus and doing their best to avoid crowds and travel that might put them at risk. Many were also wearing gloves and masks in public. "Perceived Level of Threat COVID-19 Poses to the U.S. and Individuals Doubles in Less than a Month," Ipsos, April 13, 2020, https://www.ipsos.com/sites/default/files/ct/news/documents/202004/topline_usa_today_coronavirus_w2_041320.pdf.

16. Hadas Magen, "Lockdown Lunacy: Former Health Ministry Chief Prof Yoram Lass Says Governments Can't Halt Viruses and the Lockdown Will Kill More People from Depression Than the Virus," Globes, March 22, 2020, https://en.globes.co.il/en/article-lockdown-lunacy-1001322696.

17. Jordan Schachtel (@JordanSchachtel), "So it turns out this video is entirely fraudulent," Twitter, April 6, 2020, 10:06 a.m., https://twitter.com/JordanSchachtel/status/1247163898584760320; Bernie Sanders (@SenSanders), "It is insane that our nurses are being forced to care for the sick without masks and respirators. The Department of Labor must immediately issue emergency workplace standards to protect our health workers, their families, and their patients," Twitter, April 5, 2020, 2:43 p.m., https://twitter.com/SenSanders/status/1246870982436048899.

18. Although officials designated it a COVID-19 death, his family doubts the accuracy of that designation. He died quickly without relevant symptoms, and his elderly wife showed no sign of infection.

19. For instance: Nicholas Mulder, "The Coronavirus War Economy Will Change the World," Foreign Policy, March 26, 2020, https://foreignpolicy.com/2020/03/26/the-coronavirus-war-economy-will-change-the-world.

20. Laurence Darmiento, "Charity Is off the Charts amid the Coronavirus. Is That a Sign of America's Strength or Weakness?" Los Angeles Times, April 20, 2020, https://www.latimes.com/business/story/2020-04-20/coronavirus-philanthropy-charitable-donations-inequality.

21. Chelsea Follett, "Charity Rises to the Occasion amid the Pandemic," *Human Progress*, April 8, 2020, https://humanprogress.org/article. php?p=2593.

CHAPTER 1: WHERE DID THE PANDEMIC START?

1. Franklin Delano Roosevelt, First Inaugural Address, March 4, 1933.
2. These numbers are for 2017, "Leading Causes of Death," Centers for Disease Control and Prevention, https://www.cdc.gov/nchs/fastats/ leading-causes-of-death.htm; Niki Carver, Vikas Gupta, and John E. Hipskind, "Medical Error," StatPearls, last updated May 23, 2020, https://www.ncbi.nlm.nih.gov/books/NBK430763.
3. "Coronavirus Disease 2019 (COVID-19)," Mayo Clinic, https:// www.mayoclinic.org/diseases-conditions/coronavirus/symptoms-causes/syc-20479963.
4. Jonathan Kay, "Enough with the Phony 'Lockdown' Debate," Quillette, May 8, 2020, https://quillette.com/2020/05/08/ enough-with-the-phoney-lockdown-debate.
5. Sui-Lee Wee and Vivian Wang, "China Grapples with Mystery Pneumonia-Like Illness," *New York Times*, January 6, 2020, Updated January 21, 2020, https://www.nytimes.com/2020/01/06/ world/asia/china-SARS-pneumonialike.html; Amy Qin and Javier C. Hernandez, "China Reports First Death from New Virus," *New York Times*, January 10, 2020, updated January 21, 2020, https:// www.nytimes.com/2020/01/10/world/asia/china-virus-wuhan-death. html.
6. Amy Qin and Vivian Wang, "Wuhan, Center of Coronavirus Outbreak, Is Being Cut Off by Chinese Authorities," *New York Times*, January 22, 2020, Updated January 24, 2020, https://www. nytimes.com/2020/01/22/world/asia/china-coronavirus-travel.html.
7. Donald J. Trump (@realDonaldTrump), "China has been working very hard to contain the Coronavirus. The United States greatly appreciates their efforts and transparency. It will all work out well. In particular, on behalf of the American People, I want to thank President Xi!" Twitter, January 24, 2020, 4:18 p.m., https://twitter. com/realdonaldtrump/status/1220818115354923009.
8. John McCormack, "The Senator Who Saw the Coronavirus Coming," *National Review*, March 31, 2020, https://www.nationalreview.com/2020/03/ the-senator-who-saw-the-coronavirus-coming.

9. Donald J. Trump (@realDonaldTrump), "Working closely with China and others on Coronavirus outbreak. Only 5 people in U.S., all in good recovery," Twitter, January 30, 2020, 5:04 p.m., https://twitter.com/realdonaldtrump/status/1223004106408833025.

10. Michael Corkery and Annie Karni, "Trump Administration Restricts Entry into U.S. From China," *New York Times*, January 31, 2020, Updated February 10, 2020, https://www.nytimes.com/2020/01/31/business/china-travel-coronavirus.html.

11. Dominick Mastrangelo, "Pelosi Encouraged Public Gatherings in Late February, Weeks after Trump's China Travel Ban," *Washington Examiner*, March 30, 2020, https://www.washingtonexaminer.com/news/pelosi-encouraged-public-gatherings-in-late-february-weeks-after-trumps-china-travel-ban.

12. A 2015 *Nature* study was the thin basis for this rumor. In 2020 the editors of the publication added a note to the article dissociating the study from the coronavirus that causes COVID-19. Declan Butler, "Engineered Bat Virus Stirs Debate over Risky Research," *Nature*, November 12, 2015, https://www.nature.com/news/engineered-bat-virus-stirs-debate-over-risky-research-1.18787.

13. "Tracking Down the Origin of Wuhan Coronavirus," Film, *The Epoch Times*, 2020, https://www.theepochtimes.com/coronavirusfilm?fbclid=IwAR2FKIEZ2RfB_awNCp64Q42mlD6qmXzyMS6CB3rm9z3BsnKSuDbJgaezGgs.

14. Junwen Luan, Yue Lu, Xiaolu Jin, and Leiliang Zhang, "Spike Protein Recognition of Mammalian ACE2 Predicts the Host Range and an Optimized ACE2 for SARS-CoV-2 Infection," *Biochemical and Biophysical Research Communications* 526, no. 1 (May 2020): 165–69, https://www.sciencedirect.com/science/article/pii/S0006291X2030526X?via%3Dihub#appsec1.

15. "E2 Glycoprotein Precursor (Severe Acute Respiratory Syndrome-Related Coronavirus)," NCBI, https://www.ncbi.nlm.nih.gov/protein/NP_828851.1.

16. "Surface Glycoprotein (Severe Acute Respiratory Syndrome Coronavirus 2)," NCBI, https://www.ncbi.nlm.nih.gov/protein/QJC20993.1.

17. "Spike Glycoprotein (Bat coronavirus RaTG13)," NCBI, https://www.ncbi.nlm.nih.gov/protein/QHR63300.

18. "Clustal Omega," EMBL-EBI, https://www.ebi.ac.uk/Tools/msa/clustalo.

19. "DDBJ Annotated/Assembled Sequences," BI-DDBJ, https://www.ddbj.nig.ac.jp/ddbj/code-e.html.

20. Nickie Louise, "Norwegian Scientist Birger Sorensen Claims Coronavirus Was Lab-Made and 'Not Natural in Origin,'" Tech Startups, June 7, 2020, https://techstartups.com/2020/06/07/norwegian-scientist-birger-sorensen-claims-coronavirus-lab-made-not-natural-origin.

21. Peter Svaar, "Norsk Forsker Skaper Strid om Virusets Opphav: – Dette Viruset Har Ikke en Naturlig Opprinnelse," NRK, last updated June 8, 2020, https://www.nrk.no/norge/norsk-forsker-skaper-strid-om-virusets-opphav_-_-dette-viruset-har-ikke-en-naturlig-opprinnelse-1.15043634.

22. B. Sørensen, A. Susrud, and A. G. Dalgleish, "Biovacc-19: A Candidate Vaccine for Covid-19 (SARS-CoV-2) Developed from Analysis of its General Method of Action for Infectivity," *QRB Discovery*, June 2020, https://www.cambridge.org/core/journals/qrb-discovery/article/biovacc19-a-candidate-vaccine-for-covid19-sarscov2-developed-from-analysis-of-its-general-method-of-action-for-infectivity/DBBC0FA6E3763B0067CAAD8F3363E527.

23. Josh Rogin, "State Department Cables Warned of Safety Issues at Wuhan Lab Studying Bat Coronaviruses," *Washington Post,* April 14, 2020, https://www.washingtonpost.com/opinions/2020/04/14/state-department-cables-warned-safety-issues-wuhan-lab-studying-bat-coronaviruses.

24. Ken Dilanian et al., "Report Says Cellphone Data Suggests October Shutdown at Wuhan Lab, but Experts Are Skeptical," NBC News, April 17, 2020, https://www.nbcnews.com/politics/national-security/report-says-cellphone-data-suggests-october-shutdown-wuhan-lab-experts-n1202716.

CHAPTER 2: WHO STARTED THE PANIC?

1. Richard Feynman, "What is Science?" *The Physics Teacher* 7, no. 6 (1969): 313–20, originally presented at the fifteenth annual meeting of the National Science Teachers Association, 1966 in New York City.

2. About WHO, World Health Organization, https://www.who.int/about.

3. "Biography of Dr. Tedros Adhanom Ghebreyesus, Director-General, World Health Organization," World Health Organization, http://www9.who.int/antimicrobial-resistance/interagency-coordination-group/dg_who_bio/en.

4. Nicholas Eberstadt and Dan Blumenthal, "China's Deadly Coronavirus-Lie Co-conspirator—the World Health Organization," *New York Post,* April 2, 2020, https://nypost.com/2020/04/02/chinas-deadly-coronavirus-lie-co-conspirator-the-world-health-organization.

5. Thanks to John Zmirak for this colorful image.

6. Kathy Gilsinan, "How China Deceived the WHO," *The Atlantic,* April 12, 2020, https://www.theatlantic.com/politics/archive/2020/04/world-health-organization-blame-pandemic-coronavirus/609820.

7. "Coronavirus Declared Global Health Emergency by WHO," BBC News, January 31, 2020, https://www.bbc.com/news/world-51318246.

8. Hong Kong World City, (@HKWORLDCITY), "!! WOW !! Bruce Aylward/@WHO did an interview with HK's @rthk_news & when asked about #Taiwan he pretended not to hear the question. The journalist asks again & he hangs up! She calls back & he said "Well, we've already talked about China." ENJOY+SHARE THE MADDNESS! #CoronaVirus," Twitter, March 28, 2020, 4:40 a.m., https://twitter.com/HKWORLDCITY/status/12438656 41448169474.

9. Jim Treacher, "WHO Expert Mysteriously Disappears from Website After Carrying Water for China," PJ Media, March 28, 2020, https://pjmedia.com/news-and-politics/jim-treacher/2020/03/28/who-expert-mysteriously-disappears-from-website-after-carrying-water-for-china-n382968. WHO said they did so to prevent the media from misidentifying him. Sure.

10. Georg Fahrion et al., "Muss Peking für die Pandemie-Schaden Zahlen?" *Spiegel Politik*, May 8, 2020, https://www.spiegel.de/politik/ausland/corona-ausbruch-vertuscht-muss-china-fuer-die-pandemie-schaeden-zahle n-a-00000000-0002-0001-0000-000170816271.

11. "15 Days to Slow the Spread," March 16, 2020, https://www.whitehouse.gov/articles/15-days-slow-spread.

12. Norman Lewis, "The Dangerous Rise of Rule by Experts," Spiked, April 28, 2020, https://www.spiked-online.com/2020/04/28/the-dangerous-rise-of-rule-by-experts.

13. Ben Peterson, "Experts, Politicians, and the Public: The Science and Art of Collective Decision-Making in a Free Society," *Public*

Discourse, April 20, 2020, https://www.thepublicdiscourse.
com/2020/04/62503.

14. Lucy Sherriff, "'A Lot of Pushback': Top Doc Fauci Admits Lives Could Have Been Saved If US Had Shut Down in February—but Recommendation 'Not Taken,'" *U.S. Sun*, April 12, 2020, https://www.the-sun.com/news/672794/fauci-lives-saved-us-shut-down-earlier.

15. "Dr. Fauci on Coronavirus Fears: No Need to Change Lifestyle Yet," *Today*, February 29, 2020, https://www.today.com/video/dr-fauci-on-coronavirus-fears-no-need-to-change-lifestyle-yet-79684677616.

16. Jeff Wise, "We Might Never Get a Good Coronavirus Vaccine," *New York Magazine*, April 20, 2020, https://nymag.com/intelligencer/2020/04/will-there-be-a-coronavirus-vaccine-maybe-not.html.

17. Debra Heine, "Fauci Walks Back Sunday Talk Show Comments about COVID-19 Mitigation Efforts," American Greatness, April 13, 2020, https://amgreatness.com/2020/04/13/fauci-walks-back-sunday-talk-show-comments-about-covid-19-mitigation-efforts.

18. Aria Bendix, "Health Experts Issued an Ominous Warning about a Coronavirus Pandemic 3 Months Ago. The Virus in Their simulation Killed 65 Million People," *Business Insider*, January 23, 2020, https://www.businessinsider.com/scientist-simulated-coronavirus-pandemic-deaths-2020-1; John Koetsier, "AI Predicts Coronavirus Could Infect 2.5 Billion and Kill 53 Million. Doctors Say That's Not Credible, And Here's Why," *Forbes*, February 5, 2020, https://www.forbes.com/sites/johnkoetsier/2020/02/05/ai-predicts-coronavirus-could-infect-25b-and-kill-53m-doctors-say-thats-not-credible-and-heres-why/#15a43c5e11cd; Patrick Knox, "Apocalypse Now. Bill Gates 'Predicted' How Coronavirus-Like Pandemic Could Spread Saying 33 MILLION May Die in First Six Months," *U.S. Sun*, January 24, 2020, https://www.the-sun.com/news/306110/bill-gates-predicted-chinese-coronavirus-a-year-ago-as-simulation-suggests-65-million-could-die; Fabienne Lang, "An 'IT Person' Predicted How Many Deaths the Coronavirus Will Really Cause," Interesting Engineering, February 4, 2020, https://interestingengineering.com/an-it-person-predicted-how-many-deaths-the-coronavirus-will-really-cause; Michael Le Page and Debora Mackenzie, "Could the New

Coronavirus Really Kill 50 Million People Worldwide?" *New Scientist*, February 11, 2020, https://www.newscientist.com/article/2233085-could-the-new-coronavirus-really-kill-50-million-people-worldwide.

19. Eliza Barclay and Dylan Scott, "How Canceled Events and Self-Quarantines Save Lives, in One Chart," Vox, March 10, 2020, https://www.vox.com/2020/3/10/21171481/coronavirus-us-cases-quarantine-cancellation; Barack Obama (@BarackObama), "If you're wondering whether it's an overreaction to cancel large gatherings and public events (and I love basketball), here's a useful primer as to why these measures can slow the spread of the virus and save lives. We have to look out for each other," Twitter, March 12, 2020, 7:00 p.m., https://twitter.com/BarackObama/status/1238238576141352966.

20. Brandin Specktor, "Coronavirus: What Is 'Flattening the Curve,' and Will It Work?" Live Science, March 16, 2020, https://www.livescience.com/coronavirus-flatten-the-curve.html.

21. Heather Mongilio and Jeremy Arias, "Stay-at-Home Order Announced in Maryland; Policing Seeing Compliance," *Frederick News-Post*, March 20, 2020, https://www.fredericknewspost.com/news/continuing_coverage/coronavirus/stay-at-home-order-announced-in-maryland-police-seeing-compliance/article_4a7bd963-c3ce-5731-8c45-8617e9dad410.html.

22. "COVID-19 Public Health Response Bill," New Zealand Legislation, May 12, 2020, http://www.legislation.govt.nz/bill/government/2020/0246/latest/LMS344194.html.

23. "CDC Activities and Initiatives Supporting the COVID-19 Response and the President's Plan for Opening America Up Again," CDC, May 2020, https://www.cdc.gov/coronavirus/2019-ncov/downloads/php/CDC-Activities-Initiatives-for-COVID-19-Response.pdf.

CHAPTER 3: HOW IT SPREAD

1. Evita Ochel, "The Fearmongering Stops Here. The Solutions Start with You," Evolving Beings, April 10, 2020, https://www.evolvingbeings.com/post/the-fearmongering-stops-here-the-solutions-start-with-you.

2. Holman W. Jenkins Jr., "The Media vs. Flatten the Curve," *Wall Street Journal*, April 28, 2020, https://www.wsj.com/articles/the-media-vs-flatten-the-curve-11588113213.

3.   Rong-Gong Lin II and Sean Greene, "Californians are Losing Their Fear of the Coronavirus, Setting the Stage for Disaster," *Los Angeles Times,* July 3, 2020, https://www.latimes.com/california/story/2020-07-03/how-california-went-from-coronavirus-success-story-to-sitting-on-the-precipice-of-disaster.

4.   Estimated infection rates are from the CDC. See, for example, "CDC Says COVID-19 Cases in U.S. May be 10 Times Higher Than Reported," NBC News, June 26, 2020, https://www.nbcnews.com/health/health-news/cdc-says-covid-19-cases-u-s-may-be-10-n1232134.

5.   Consider the Diamond Princess cruise ship, which had 2,670 passengers and 1,110 crew, which went under forced quarantine. Yet only 712 persons (19 percent) became infected. "COVID-19 CORONAVIRUS PANDEMIC," Worldometer, last updated July 21, 2020, https://www.worldometers.info/coronavirus.

6.   Maxford Nelsen, "Washington State Over-Reporting COVID-19 Deaths," Freedom Foundation, May 18, 2020, https://www.freedomfoundation.com/washington/washington-state-over-reporting-covid-19-deaths.

7.   Maxford Nelsen, "Washington Health Officials: Gunshot Victims Counted as COVID-19 Deaths," *Freedom Foundation*, May 21, 2020, https://www.freedomfoundation.com/washington/washington-health-officials-gunshot-victims-counted-as-covid-19-deaths.

8.   "New York City Posts Sharp Spike in Coronavirus Deaths After Untested Victims Added," Reuters, April 14, 2020, https://www.reuters.com/article/us-health-coronavirus-usa/new-york-city-posts-sharp-spike-in-coronavirus-deaths-after-untested-victims-added-idUSKCN21W20G.

9.   This is revealed by plotting the number of tests and new positive cases, which shows a strong linear relationship in most locations.

10. Emma Keith, "Oklahoma Reports 222 New COVID-19 Cases, 6 in Cleveland County," *Norman Transcript,* June 12, 2020, https://www.normantranscript.com/news/oklahoma-reports-222-new-covid-19-cases-6-in-cleveland-county/article_8040441a-acca-11ea-9fc2-7f4719c4166e.html.

11. Darla Shelden, "CVS Announces New Oklahoma Site for Free COVID-19 Testing," *City Sentinel,* June 19, 2020, http://city-sentinel.com/2020/06/cvs-announces-new-oklahoma-site-for-free-covid-19-testing.

12. "More than Half of Oklahoma's COVID-19 Cases Confirmed in June, According to OSDH Data," *Enid New & Eagle*, July 1, 2020, https://www.enidnews.com/news/covid19/over-half-of-oklahomas-covid-19-cases-confirmed-in-june-according-to-osdh-data/article_bc503fb4-bbb6-11ea-a9e5-4bed3730bc7c.html.

13. United States COVID-19 Statistics, https://covidusa.net.

14. "Initial COVID-19 Infection Rate May Be 80 Times Greater Than Originally Reported," *Penn State News*, July 2, 2020, https://news.psu.edu/story/623797/2020/06/22/research/initial-covid-19-infection-rate-may-be-80-times-greater-originally.

15. Phillip Zucs et al., "Influenza Associated Excess Mortality in Germany, 1985–2001," *Emerging Themes in Epidemiology* 2, no. 6 (June 2005): 1–9, https://ete-online.biomedcentral.com/articles/10.1186/1742-7622-2-6.

16. "Deaths from Pneumonia and Influenza," CDC, https://data.cdc.gov/Health-Statistics/Deaths-from-Pneumonia-and-Influenza-P-I-and-all-de/pp7x-dyj2/dat.

17. "Burden of Influenza," CDC, https://www.cdc.gov/flu/about/burden/index.html.

18. Ari Schulman, Brendan Foht, and Samuel Matlack, "Not Like the Flu, Not Like Car Crashes, Not Like…It's about the Spike," *New Atlantis*, May 19, 2020, https://www.thenewatlantis.com/publications/not-like-the-flu-not-like-car-crashes-not-like.

19. "1957–1958 Pandemic (H2N2 virus)," CDC, https://www.cdc.gov/flu/pandemic-resources/1957-1958-pandemic.html.

20. As of June 30, 2020, Worldometer (which tends to overcount) had global deaths from COVID-19 at 409,708, https://www.worldometers.info/coronavirus.

21. Schulman, Foht, and Matlack, "Not like the Flu."

22. Ibid.

23. Real Time with Billy Maher, "New Rule: Panic Porn," YouTube video, April 17, 2020, https://www.youtube.com/watch?time_continue=8&v=UcvIQJ-QurQ&feature=emb_logo.

CHAPTER 4: SOCIAL MANIAS AND THE CULT OF EXPERTISE

1. Glenn Greenwald, Goodreads, http://www.goodreads.com/quotes/426096-incestuous-homogeneous-fiefdoms-of-self-proclaimed- expertise-are-always-rank-closing-and.

2. Garrett M. Graff, "Experts Knew a Pandemic Was Coming. Here's What They're Worried About Next," *Politico*, May 7, 2020, https://www.politico.com/news/magazine/2020/05/07/experts-knew-pandemic-was-coming-what-they-fear-next-238686.

3. "Smartphone Penetration in the United States from 2008 to 2014," Statista, January 10, 2012, https://www.statista.com/statistics/218529/us-martphone-penetration-since-2008.

4. "With Smartphone Adoption on the Rise, Opportunity for Marketers is Calling," Nielsen, September 15, 2009, https://www.nielsen.com/us/en/insights/article/2009/with-smartphone-adoption-on-the-rise-opportunity-for-marketers-is-calling.

5. "Smartphone Ownership Rate by Country 2018," Statista, February 27, 2020, https://www.statista.com/statistics/539395/smartphone-penetration-worldwide-by-country.

6. "How Many People Have Smartphones in 2020?" Oberlo, https://www.oberlo.com/statistics/how-many-people-have-smartphones.

7. Mansoor Iqbal, "WhatsApp Revenue and Usage Statistics (2020)," Business of Apps, June 23, 2020, https://www.businessofapps.com/data/whatsapp-statistics.

8. Mercedes Bunz, "Has Twitter Reached Its Peak?" *The Guardian*, March 12, 2010, https://www.theguardian.com/media/pda/2010/mar/12/twitter-growth.

9. Ying Lin, "10 Twitter Statistics Every Marketer Should Know in 2020," Oberlo, November 30, 2019, https://www.oberlo.com/blog/twitter-statistics.

10. "Timeline of Instagram," Wikipedia, last updated June 18, 2020, https://en.wikipedia.org/wiki/Timeline_of_Instagram.

11. "Instagram by the Numbers: Stats, Demographics & Fun Facts," Omnicore, February 10, 2020, https://www.omnicoreagency.com/instagram-statistics.

12. "Number of Active Users at Facebook Over the Years," Finance, October 23, 2012, https://finance.yahoo.com/news/number-active-users-facebook-over-years-214600186—finance.html.

13. J. Clement, "Number of Facebook Users Worldwide From 2015 to 2020," Statista, November 15, 2019, https://www.statista.com/statistics/490424/number-of-worldwide-facebook-users.

14. Mansoor Iqbal, "YouTube Revenue and Usage Statistics (2020)," Business of Apps, June 23, 2020, https://www.businessofapps.com/data/youtube-statistics.

15. Robert M. Metcalfe, "It's All in Your Head," *Forbes*, April 20, 2007, https://www.forbes.com/forbes/2007/0507/052.html#4e1cbf5347d3.
16. Raheem Kassam (@RaheemKassam), "YouTube CEO @ SusanWojcicki says they'll censor vids not approved by Tedros's @ WHO. 1. Tedros is a CCP supporter, covered up cholera outbreaks. 2: WHO has recommended "traditional Chinese medicine". 3: WHO had Mugabe as a 'goodwill ambassador'. Not the best company, Suze," Twitter, April 21, 2020, 6:11 p.m., https://twitter.com/ RaheemKassam/status/1252721653240528896. YouTube was also caught, in May, deleting comments to all videos containing phrases said to be "insulting" to China's Communist Party. See James Vincent, "YouTube Is Deleting Comments with Two Phrases That Insult China's Communist Party," The Verge, May 26, 2020, https:// www.theverge.com/2020/5/26/21270290/youtube-deleting-comments-censorship-chinese-communist-party-ccp.
17. Veronica Morley, "Accelerated Urgent Care Doctors Recommend Lifting Shelter-in-Place Order," 23ABC News Bakersfield, April 22, 2020, https://www.turnto23.com/news/coronavirus/ accelerated-urgent-care-doctors-recommend-lifting-shelter-in-place-order.
18. Eliza Relman, "Facebook Is Removing Promotions for Anti-Quarantine Protests That Violate Stay-Home Orders in California, New Jersey, and Nebraska," *Business Insider*, April 20, 2020, https:// www.businessinsider.com/coronavirus-facebook-is-removing-promotions-for-anti-quarantine-protests-2020-4.
19. Justin P. Hicks, "Facebook Deletes Event for Stay-at-Home Protest in Michigan," Michigan Live, April 29, 2020, https://www.mlive.com/ public-interest/2020/04/facebook-deletes-event-for-stay-at-home-protest-in-michigan.html.
20. Jon Levine, "YouTube Censors Epidemiologist Knut Wittkowski for Opposing Lockdown," *New York Post*, May 16, 2020, https:// nypost.com/2020/05/16/ youtube-censors-epidemiologist-knut-wittkowski-for-opposing-lockdown.
21. "The Rockefeller University Releases Statement Concerning Knut Wittkowski," The Rockefeller University, April 13, 2020, https:// www.rockefeller.edu/news/27872-rockefeller-university-releases-statement-concerning-dr-knut-wittkowski.

22. "Our Story," Heterodox Academy, https://heterodoxacademy.org/our-story.

23. Kate Starbird, Emma Spiro, and Jevin West, "This Covid-19 Misinformation Went Viral: Here's What We Learned," *Washington Post*, May 8, 2020, https://www.washingtonpost.com/politics/2020/05/08/this-covid-19-misinformation-went-viral-heres-what-we-learned.

24. Zoe Schiffer, "How Medium Became the Best and Worst Place for Coronavirus News," *The Verge*, April 14, 2020, https://www.theverge.com/2020/4/14/21219907/medium-coronavirus-covid-19-news-misinformation-conspiracy-theories-best-worst.

25. Eran Bendavid et al., "COVID-19 Antibody Seroprevalence in Santa Clara County, California," MedRxiv, April 30, 2020, https://www.medrxiv.org/content/10.1101/2020.04.14.20062463v2.

26. Aleszu Bajak and Jeff Howe, "A Study Said Covid Wasn't That Deadly. The Right Seized It," *New York Times*, May 14, 2020, https://www.nytimes.com/2020/05/14/opinion/coronavirus-research-misinformation.html.

27. Marc Lipsitch (@mlipsitch), "It's getting increasingly hard to take John Ioannidis's 'let's keep to the science' line seriously. My postdoc advisor Bruce Levin said 'What distinguishes science from the rest of academia is that in science, you can't predict the conclusion from the name of the author,'" Twitter, May 20, 2020, 10:34 p.m., https://twitter.com/mlipsitch/status/1263296963627356161.

28. Jeet Heer, "How Stanford Lost its Soul," *The Nation*, May 20, 2020, https://www.thenation.com/article/society/stanford-lost-soul-coronavirus.

29. Josephine Moulds, "How Is the World Health Organization Funded?" World Economic Forum, April 15, 2020, https://www.weforum.org/agenda/2020/04/who-funds-world-health-organization-un-coronavirus-pandemic-covid-trump.

CHAPTER 5: RUSH TO LOCKDOWN

1. H. L. Mencken, *A Little Book in C Major* (New York: John Lane Co., 1916).

2. Frank Newport, "10 Key Findings: Public Opinion on Coronavirus," Gallup, March 20, 2020, https://news.gallup.com/opinion/polling-matters/296681/ten-key-findings-public-opinion-coronavirus.aspx.

3. Christina Capatides, "'Shoot Them Dead': Philippine President Rodrigo Duterte Orders Police and Military to Kill Citizens Who Defy Coronavirus Lockdown," CBS News, April 2, 2020, https://www.cbsnews.com/news/rodrigo-duterte-philippines-president-coronavirus-lockdown-shoot-people-dead.

4. Ankita Mukhopadhyay, "India: Police under Fire for Using Violence to Enforce Coronavirus Lockdown," Deutsche Welle, March 28, 2020, https://www.dw.com/en/india-police-under-fire-for-using-violence-to-enforce-coronavirus-lockdown/a-52946717.

5. Steven Nelson, "DC Mayor Threatens Jail Time for Leaving Home during Coronavirus," *New York Post*, March 30, 2020, https://nypost.com/2020/03/30/dc-mayor-threatens-jail-time-for-leaving-home-during-coronavirus.

6. Wilson Ring and Travis Pittman, "Vermont Orders Walmart, Target to Stop Selling Non-Essential Items in the Store," 13 WTHR, April 2, 2020, last updated April 3, 2020, https://www.wthr.com/article/vermont-orders-walmart-target-stop-selling-non-essential-items-store.

7. Brendan O'Neill, "The Sickness of Snitching," Spiked, March 30, 2020, https://www.spiked-online.com/2020/03/30/the-sickness-of-snitching.

8. Madeline Chambers, "Germans Snitch on Neighbours Flouting Virus Rules, in Echo of the Stasi Past," Thomson Reuters Foundation News, April 2, 2020, https://news.trust.org/item/20200402160625-8y12u.

9. "Taipei City Government to Reward Those Who Report Mask Litterers," *Taiwan News*, April 2, 2020, https://www.taiwannews.com.tw/en/news/3909264.

10. "'Snitches Get Rewards': Garcetti Issues New Rules for Construction Sites, Encourages Community to Report Safer at Home Violators," CBS Los Angeles, March 31, 2020, https://losangeles.cbslocal.com/2020/03/31/coronavirus-los-angeles-eric-garcetti-snitches-get-rewards.

11. "Coronavirus Delaware: Police Authorized to Pull Over Out-of-State Drivers during Pandemic," 3 CBS Philly, April 2, 2020, https://

philadelphia.cbslocal.com/2020/04/02/
coronavirus-delaware-police-authorized-to-pull-over-out-of-state-
drivers-during-pandemic.

12. "Remarks by President Trump, Vice President Pence, and Members of
the Coronavirus Task Force in Press Briefing," White House, March
31, 2020, https://www.whitehouse.gov/briefings-statements/
remarks-president-trump-vice-president-pence-members-coronavirus-
task-force-press-briefing-15.

13. Ted Cruz, "Ted Cruz: Social-Distancing Restrictions Are Fine—Petty
Authoritarianism Is Not," *New York Post*, April 14, 2020, https://
nypost.com/2020/04/14/ted-cruz-social-distancing-restrictions-
are-fine-petty-authoritarianism-is-not.

14. "Why Do People Hoard and Socialize during a Pandemic?"
University of Rochester, April 2, 2020, https://www.rochester.edu/
newscenter/covid-19-hoard-socialize-pandemic-421442.

15. Thomas Joseph White, "Epidemic Danger and Catholic Sacraments,"
First Things, April 4, 2020, https://www.firstthings.com/web-
exclusives/2020/04/epidemic-danger-and-catholic-sacraments.

16. Toluse Olorunnipa, Shawn Boburg, and Arelis R. Hernandez,
"Rallies against Stay-at-Home Orders Grow as Trump Sides with
Protesters," *Washington Post*, April 17, 2020, https://www.
washingtonpost.com/national/rallies-against-stay-at-home-orders-
grow-as-trump-sides-with-protesters/2020/04/17/1405ba54-7f4e-
11ea-8013-1b6da0e4a2b7_story.html.

17. Mark Harris (@MarkHarrisNYC), "I'll never forget the day Rosa
Parks got on the bus with a submachine gun and refused to wear a
mask because of freedom," Twitter, April 18, 2020, 1:31 p.m., https://
twitter.com/MarkHarrisNYC/status/1251563951864852480.

CHAPTER 6: UNTANGLING THE NUMBERS

1. Timothy Akinyomi, "If You Torture the Data Long Enough, It Will
Confess to Anything," Business Day, January 29, 2020, https://
businessday.ng/opinion/article/if-you-torture-the-data-long-enough-it-
will-confess-to-anything/amp.

2. "Statement on the Second Meeting of the International Health
Regulations (2005) Emergency Committee Regarding the Outbreak
of Novel Coronavirus (2019-nCoV)," World Health Organization,
January 30, 2020, https://www.who.int/news-room/
detail/30-01-2020-statement-on-the-second-meeting-of-the-

international-health-regulations-(2005)-emergency-committee-regarding-the-outbreak-of-novel-coronavirus-(2019-ncov).

3. "WHO Director-General's Opening Remarks at the Media Briefing on COVID-19," World Health Organization, March 11, 2020, https://www.who.int/dg/speeches/detail/who-director-general-s-opening-remarks-at-the-media-briefing-on-covid-19---11-march-2020.

4. "COVID-19 Coding in ICD-10," World Health Organization, March 25, 2020, https://www.who.int/classifications/icd/COVID-19-coding-icd10.pdf?ua=1.

5. "Emergency Use ICD Codes for COVID-19 Disease Outbreak," World Health Organization, https://www.who.int/classifications/icd/covid19/en.

6. "Total Number of COVID-19 Tests per Confirmed Case," Our World in Data, April 19, 2020, https://ourworldindata.org/grapher/number-of-covid-19-tests-per-confirmed-case?time=2020-04-19.

7. Deaths are coded to U07.1 when coronavirus disease 2019 or COVID-19 are reported as a cause that contributed to death on the death certificate. These can include laboratory confirmed cases, as well as cases without laboratory confirmation. "Daily Updates of Totals by Week and State: Provisional Death Counts for Coronavirus Disease 2019," CDC, April 6, 2020, https://www.cdc.gov/nchs/nvss/vsrr/COVID19/index.htm. This contradicts the WHO protocol cited in note 2 to this chapter, above.

8. "Daily New Deaths in the United States," Worldometer, last updated July 26, 2020, https://www.worldometers.info/coronavirus/country/us.

9. "Sad, Angry, and Confused: Family Says Mother Was Never Tested, but Death Certificate Lists COVID-19," WHEC TV, May 21, 2020, https://www.whec.com/coronavirus/mother-was-never-tested-but-death-certificate-lists-covid-19/5737087.

10. "Daily Updates of Totals by Week and State: Provisional Death Counts for Coronavirus Disease 2019," CDC, July 2, 2020, https://www.cdc.gov/nchs/nvss/vsrr/COVID19/index.htm.

11. John Lee, "How Deadly Is the Coronavirus? It's Still Far from Clear," *Spectator*, March 28, 2020, https://www.spectator.co.uk/article/The-evidence-on-Covid-19-is-not-as-clear-as-we-think.

12. Bob Brigham, "Deborah Birx Reportedly Tells Task Force She Can Trust 'Nothing from the CDC,'" Salon, May 9, 2020, https://www.

salon.com/2020/05/09/
deborah-birx-reportedly-tells-task-force-she-can-trust-nothing-from-
the-cdc_partner.

13. Frauke Rudolf et al., "Influence of Referral Pathway on Ebola Virus
Disease Case-Fatality Rate and Effect of Survival Selection Bias,"
Emerging Infectious Diseases 23, no. 4 (April 2017): 597–600,
https://www.ncbi.nlm.nih.gov/pubmed/28322693.

14. Jordi Rello and Aurora Pop-Vicas, "Clinical Review: Primary
Influenza Viral Pneumonia," *Critical Care* 13, no. 6 (December
2009): 235, https://www.ncbi.nlm.nih.gov/pmc/articles/
PMC2811908.

15. Ibid.

16. "2009 H1N1 Early Outbreak and Disease Characteristics," CDC,
October 27, 2009, https://www.cdc.gov/h1n1flu/surveillanceqa.htm.

17. "Division of Vital Statistics, Mortality Data," CDC, March 17, 2016,
https://www.cdc.gov/nchs/data/health_policy/influenza-and-
pneumonia-deaths-2008-2015.pdf.

18. Grant W. Waterer et al., "In-Hospital Deaths Among Adults with
Community-Acquired Pneumonia," *Chest* 154, no. 3 (September
2018): 628–35, https://journal.chestnet.org/article/S0012-
3692(18)30801-8/fulltext.

19. Ibid.

20. Graziano Onder, Giovanni Ressa, and Silvio Brusaferro, "Case-
Fatality Rate and Characteristics of Patients Dying in Relation to
COVID-19 in Italy," *Journal of the American Medical Association*
323, no. 18 (March 2020): 1775–76, https://jamanetwork.com/
journals/jama/fullarticle/2763667.

21. "Weekly Updates by Select Demographic and Geographic
Characteristics: Provisional Death Counts for Coronavirus Disease
(COVID-19); Table 2c," CDC, May 20, 2020, https://www.cdc.gov/
nchs/nvss/vsrr/covid_weekly/index.htm#AgeAndSex.

22. "Fatalities," New York State Department of Health, last updated July
27, 2020, https://covid19tracker.health.ny.gov/views/NYS-COVID19-
Tracker/NYSDOHCOVID-19Tracker-Fatalities?%3Aembed=yes&
%3Atoolbar=no&%3Atabs=n#/views.

23. Karen Yourish et al., "One-Third of All U.S. Coronavirus Deaths Are
Nursing Home Residents or Workers," *New York Times*, May 11,
2020, https://www.nytimes.com/interactive/2020/05/09/us/
coronavirus-cases-nursing-homes-us.html.

24. "Weekly Updates by Select Demographic and Geographic Characteristics: Provisional Death Counts for Coronavirus Disease (COVID-19); Table 4," CDC, May 20, 2020, https://www.cdc.gov/nchs/nvss/vsrr/covid_weekly/index.htm#AgeAndSex.

25. "The COVID Tracking Project," The COVID Tracking Project: *The Atlantic*, https://covidtracking.com/api.

26. "Pneumonia and Influenza Mortality Surveillance from the National Center for Health Statistics Mortality Surveillance System," CDC, https://gis.cdc.gov/grasp/fluview/mortality.html.

27. "Texas Faces a Spike in the Coronavirus Cases at Meatpacking Plants," NPR, May 18, 2020, https://www.npr.org/2020/05/18/858236538/texas-faces-a-spike-in-the-coronavirus-cases-at-meatpacking-plants.

28. Peter Sullivan, "Texas, North Carolina, Arizona See Rising Cases As They Reopen," *The Hill*, May 19, 2020, https://thehill.com/policy/healthcare/498406-texas-north-carolina-arizona-see-rising-cases-as-they-reopen.

29. See, for example, "California Coronavirus Surged Tied to Increase in Testing, Not Reopening Businesses, Official Says," *Los Angeles Times*, June 13, 2020, https://www.latimes.com/california/story/2020-06-13/california-coronavirus-surge-tied-to-testing-not-reopening-businesses-officials-say.

30. Anirban Basu, "Estimating the Infection Fatality Rate among Symptomatic COVID-19 Cases in the United States," *Health Affairs*, May 7, 2020, https://www.healthaffairs.org/doi/full/10.1377/hlthaff.2020.00455.

31. Dimple D Rajgor, et al., "The Many Estimates of the COVID-19 Case Fatality Rate," *Lancet*, March 27, 2020, https://www.thelancet.com/pdfs/journals/laninf/PIIS1473-3099(20)30244-9.pdf?fbclid=IwAR0X5ZxmhzdVUC5Uas_GYlAtpQlX7K0BVg39h3EcnnRh46MBRGjHoyxw3WY.

32. Jaffar A. Al-Tawfiq, "Asymptomatic Coronavirus Infection: MERS-CoV and SARS-CoV-2 (COVID-19)," *Travel Medicine and Infectious Disease*, (February 2020), https://library.umsu.ac.ir/uploads/25_1481_51_71.pdf.

33. Justin Fox, "The Coronavirus Isn't Just the Flu, Bro," Bloomberg, April 24, 2020, https://www.bloomberg.com/opinion/articles/2020-04-24/is-coronavirus-worse-than-the-flu-blood-studies-

say-yes-by-far; Rachael Rettner, "How Does the New Coronavirus Compare with the Flu?" Live Science, May 2020, https://www.livescience.com/new-coronavirus-compare-with-flu.html.

34. Steven Riley et al., "Epidemiological Characteristics of 2009 (H1N1) Pandemic Influenza Based on Paired Sera from a Longitudinal Community Cohort Study," PLOS Medicine 8, no. 6 (June 2011): e1000442, https://www.ncbi.nlm.nih.gov/pmc/articles/PMC3119689.

35. "Pandemic Planning Scenarios," CDC, last updated July 10, 2020, https://www.cdc.gov/coronavirus/2019-ncov/hcp/planning-scenarios.html; Also see Daniel Horowitz, "The CDC Confirms Remarkably Low Coronavirus Death Rate. Where Is the Media?" Ron Paul Institute for Peace and Prosperity, May 24, 2020, http://ronpaulinstitute.org/archives/featured-articles/2020/may/24/the-cdc-confirms-remarkably-low-coronavirus-death-rate-where-is-the-media.

36. "No 'Nosocomial Infection' with 112 Cruise Ship Treatments! Why 'Self-Defense Force Central Hospital' Could Make a Miracle," Daily Shincho, April 30, 2020, https://www.dailyshincho.jp/article/2020/04300801/?all=1.

37. "List of Epidemics," Wikipedia, last updated July 26, 2020, https://en.wikipedia.org/wiki/List_of_epidemics.

38. "Out in the Cold and Back: New-Found Interest in the Great Flu," Cultural and Social History 3, no. 4 (October 2006): 496–505, https://www.researchgate.net/publication/233523876_Out_in_the_Cold_and_Back_New-Found_Interest_in_the_Great_Flu.

39. This choice shows a so-called measurement availability bias. We know far more about modern than ancient pandemics. We lack detailed records from earlier times. Our ancestors took death more for granted than we do. We moderns also fixate on precise numbers. Clusters of a few dozen deaths are now "breaking news." Centuries ago, scribes recorded only the largest outbreaks.

40. "World Population," Wikipedia, last updated July 21, 2020, https://en.wikipedia.org/wiki/World_population.

41. "Up to 650,000 People Die of Respiratory Diseases Linked to Seasonal Flu Each Year," World Health Organization, December 14, 2017, https://www.who.int/news-room/detail/14-12-2017-up-to-650-000-people-die-of-respiratory-diseases-linked-to-seasonal-flu-each-year.

42. "Weekly U.S. Influenza Surveillance Report (FluView)," CDC, last updated July 24, 2020, https://www.cdc.gov/flu/weekly.

43. "Burden of Influenza," CDC, last updated April 17, 2020, https://www.cdc.gov/flu/about/burden/index.html.

44. "2019–2020 U.S. Flu Season: Preliminary Burden Estimates," CDC, last updated April 17, 2020, https://www.cdc.gov/flu/about/burden/preliminary-in-season-estimates.htm.

45. There is evidence that the media downplayed the swine flu. See Chrissy Clark, "CNN Downplayed Swine Flu Under Obama, Went Gonzo on Wuhan Flu Under Trump," The Federalist, March 19, 2020, https://thefederalist.com/2020/03/19/cnn-downplayed-swine-flu-under-obama-went-gonzo-on-wuhan-flu-under-trump.

46. Leo Shane III, "Biden, Sanders Say Military Could Play a Role in Coronavirus Response," Military Times, March 15, 2020, https://www.militarytimes.com/news/pentagon-congress/2020/03/16/biden-sanders-say-military-could-play-a-role-in-coronavirus-response.

CHAPTER 7: BLIND MODELS

1. Story told by Charles Murray in *Human Diversity: The Biology of Gender, Race, and Class* (New York: Twelve, 2020).

2. Jonathan Ford, "The Battle at the Heart of British Science over Coronavirus," *Financial Times*, April 15, 2020, https://www.ft.com/content/1e390ac6-7e2c-11ea-8fdb-7ec06edeef84.

3. Steerpike, "Six Questions that Neil Ferguson Should Be Asked," *Spectator*, April 16, 2020, https://www.spectator.co.uk/article/six-questions-that-neil-ferguson-should-be-asked.

4. Lee Elliot Major, "BSE-Infected Sheep a 'Greater Risk' to Humans," *The Guardian*, January 9, 2002,https://www.theguardian.com/education/2002/jan/09/research.highereducation.

5. James Sturcke, "Bird Flu Pandemic 'Could Kill 150m,'" *The Guardian*, September 30, 2005, https://www.theguardian.com/world/2005/sep/30/birdflu.jamessturcke.

6. "WHO H5N1 Mortality Report", March 31, 2015, https://www.who.int/influenza/human_animal_interface/EN_GIP_201503031cumulativeNumberH5N1cases.pdf.

7. Ibid.

8. Ford, "The Battle at the Heart of British Science."

9. Max Roser, "The Spanish Flu (1918–20): The Global Impact of the Largest Influenza Pandemic in History," Our World in Data, March 4, 2020, https://ourworldindata.org/spanish-flu-largest-influenza-pandemic-in-history.

10. Sabine L. van Elsland and Ryan O'Hare, "Coronavirus Pandemic Could Have Caused 40 Million Deaths If Left Unchecked," Imperial College London News, March 26, 2020, https://www.imperial.ac.uk/news/196496/coronavirus-pandemic-could-have-caused-40.

11. Neil Ferguson et al., "Report 9: Impact of Non-Pharmaceutical Interventions (NPIs) to Reduce COVID-19 Mortality and Healthcare Demand," Imperial College London News, March 16, 2020, https://www.imperial.ac.uk/media/imperial-college/medicine/mrc-gida/2020-03-16-COVID19-Report-9.pdf.

12. Sabine L. van Elsland and Ryan O'Hare, "Coronavirus Pandemic Could Have Caused 40 Million Deaths if Left Unchecked," Imperial College London News, March 26, 2020, https://www.imperial.ac.uk/news/196496/coronavirus-pandemic-could-have-caused-40.

13. Philippe Lemoine (@phl43), "Many people claim that, if the ICL model wildly overestimated how bad the epidemic would be in Sweden without a lockdown (https://medrxiv.org/content/10.1101/20 20.04.11.20062133v1…), it's just because it didn't take into account voluntary social distancing, but I have some bad news for them," Twitter, May 21, 2020, 11:51 a.m., https://twitter.com/phl43/status/1263497666144669696.

14. "Sweden," Worldometer, last updated July 28, 2020, https://www.worldometers.info/coronavirus/country/sweden.

15. "Should We Pay the Rainmaker?" History Nebraska, https://history.nebraska.gov/publications/should-we-pay-rainmaker.

16. J. R. Stone, "Coronavirus Pandemic: Bakersfield Doctors Push to Lift Shelter-in-Place Order, NorCal Health Experts Disagree," ABC7, April 27, 2020, https://abc7.com/shelter-in-place-coronavirus-stay-at-home-ca/6132447.

17. Berkeley Lovelace Jr., "White House Predicts 100,000 to 240,000 Will Die in US from Coronavirus," CNBC, March 31, 2020, https://www.cnbc.com/2020/03/31/trump-says-the-coronavirus-surge-is-coming-its-going-to-be-a-very-very-painful-two-weeks.html. The model used was unspecified, but given Dr. Fauci's later comments noted below, it was likely the Institute for Health Metrics and Evaluation model.

18. Bill Chappell, "Fauci Says U.S. Coronavirus Deaths May Be 'More Like 60,000'; Antibody Tests On Way," NPR, April 9, 2020, https://www.npr.org/2020/04/09/830664814/fauci-says-u-s-coronavirus-deaths-may-be-more-like-60-000-antibody-tests-on-way.

19. Ibid.

20. Katherine Shaver and John D. Harden, "Most of Us Are under Stay-at-Home Orders. So Why Are 6 out of 10 Vehicles Still on the Road?" *Washington Post*, April 4, 2020, https://www.washingtonpost.com/local/trafficandcommuting/most-of-us-are-under-stay-at-home-orders-so-why-are-6-out-of-10-still-on-the-road/2020/04/04/162adcc6-7434-11ea-87da-77a8136c1a6d_story.html; Sean McMinn, "Mobile Phone Data Show More Americans Are Leaving Their Homes, Despite Orders," NPR, May 1, 2020, https://www.npr.org/2020/05/01/849161820/mobile-phone-data-show-more-americans-are-leaving-their-homes-despite-orders.

21. "Coronavirus Impact: Updated Model Predicts COVID-19 Peak in Late-July With SAHO Extended through May; 25K Deaths Possible," CBS Minnesota, May 11, 2020, https://minnesota.cbslocal.com/2020/05/11/coronavirus-impact-updated-model-predicts-covid-19-peak-in-late-july-with-saho-extended-through-may-25k-deaths-possible.

22. Ibid.

23. "SARS-CoV-2 (COVID-19) Modeling (Version 2.0)," Minnesota Department of Health, April 28, 2020, https://mn.gov/covid19/assets/MNmodel_PPT_FINAL%204.10.20_revised%2020200501_tcm1148-430665.pdf.

24. Ferguson et al., "Report 9."

25. David Adam, "Special Report: The Simulations Driving the World's Response to COVID-19. How Epidemiologists Rushed to Model the Coronavirus Pandemic," *Nature*, April 3, 2020, https://www.nature.com/articles/d41586-020-01003-6.

26. Sue Denim (pseudonym lol), "Code Review of Ferguson's Model," Lockdown Sceptics, May 10, 2020, https://lockdownsceptics.org/code-review-of-fergusons-model.

27. Ibid. The critique actually centered on R0, which is the initial value of R_e in a susceptible population.

28. Adam, "Special Report: The Simulations Driving the World's Response."

29. David Richards and Konstantin Boudnik, "Neil Ferguson's Imperial Model Could Be the Most Devastating Software Mistake of All Time," *Telegraph*, May 16, 2020, https://www.telegraph.co.uk/technology/2020/05/16/neil-fergusons-imperial-model-could-devastating-software-mistake.

30. Hannah Boland and Ellie Zolfagharifard, "Coding That Led to Lockdown Was 'Totally Unreliable' and a 'Buggy Mess', Say Experts," *Telegraph*, May 16, 2020, https://www.telegraph.co.uk/technology/2020/05/16/coding-led-lockdown-totally-unreliable-buggy-mess-say-experts.

31. "Report 9: Impact of Non-Pharmaceutical Interventions (NPIs) to Reduce COVID-19 Mortality and Healthcare Demand," Imperial College COVID-19 Response Team, March 16, 2020, https://www.imperial.ac.uk/media/imperial-college/medicine/sph/ide/gida-fellowships/Imperial-College-COVID19-NPI-modelling-16-03-2020.pdf.

32. Ibid.

33. Max Roser, "The Spanish Flu (1918–20): The Global Impact of the Largest Influenza Pandemic in History," Our World in Data, March 4, 2020, https://ourworldindata.org/spanish-flu-largest-influenza-pandemic-in-history.

34. "1918 Pandemic (H1N1 Virus)," CDC, last updated March 20, 2019, https://www.cdc.gov/flu/pandemic-resources/1918-pandemic-h1n1.html.

35. "COVID-19 Estimate Downloads," IHME, last updated July 22, 2020, http://www.healthdata.org/covid/data-downloads.

36. Ibid.

37. Eric Lipton and Jennifer Steinhauer, "The Untold Story of the Birth of Social Distancing," *New York Times*, April 22, 2020, https://www.nytimes.com/2020/04/22/us/politics/social-distancing-coronavirus.html; the co-authors of this book first read about this story in Jeffrey A. Tucker, "The 2006 Origins of the Lockdown Idea," American Institute for Economic Research, May 15, 2020, https://www.aier.org/article/the-2006-origins-of-the-lockdown-idea.; see also Robert J. Glass et al., "Targeted Social Distancing Designs for Pandemic Influenza," CDC, *Emerging Infectious Diseases* 12, no. 11

(November 2006): https://wwwnc.cdc.gov/eid/
article/12/11/06-0255_article.

38. Lipton and Steinhauer, "The Untold Story."

39. Robert J. Blendon et al., "Public Response to Community Mitigation
Measures for Pandemic Influenza," CDC, last updated July 8, 2010,
Emerging Infectious Diseases 14, no. 5 (May 2008): 778–86, https://
wwwnc.cdc.gov/eid/article/14/5/07-1437_article.

40. "The Public Engagement Project on Community Control Measures
for Pandemic Influenza," Public Policy Center, University of
Nebraska, May 2007, https://digitalcommons.unl.edu/cgi/
viewcontent.cgi?article=1106&context=publicpolicypublications.

41. Lipton and Steinhauer, "The Untold Story."

42. Scott Adams (@ScottAdamsSays), "Prediction models are not
designed to be accurate. They are designed to be useful. If you don't
understand that distinction, nothing you say about the models moves
the ball forward," Twitter, April 9, 2020, 9:32 a.m., https://twitter.
com/scottadamssays/status/1248242275781472256.

43. Ferguson et al., "Report 9," 17–18.

CHAPTER 8: WHY DID WE BELIEVE LOCKDOWNS WOULD WORK?

1. Carl Sagan, "Encyclopaedia Galactica," *Cosmos: A Personal Voyage*
(first aired on PBS December 14, 1980), Episode 12.

2. Rich Lowry, "The Absurd Case against the Coronavirus Lockdown,"
Chippewa Herald, April 18, 2020, https://chippewa.com/opinion/
columnists/rich-lowry-the-absurd-case-against-the-coronavirus-
lockdown/article_4f377a90-5e9b-5576-9456-5d90a9563ed4.html.

3. Alan Vaux and Sofia Kluch, "Americans Highly Confident Social
Distancing Saves Lives," Gallup, May 8, 2020, https://news.gallup.
com/opinion/gallup/310196/americans-highly-confident-social-
distancing-saves-lives.aspx.

4. Andrew Daniller, "Americans Remain Concerned That States Will
Lift Restrictions Too Quickly, but Partisan Differences Widen," Pew
Research Center, May 7, 2020, https://www.pewresearch.org/fact-
tank/2020/05/07/
americans-remain-concerned-that-states-will-lift-restrictions-too-
quickly-but-partisan-differences-widen.

5. Indeed, the White House and CDC campaign in March was called "15 Days to Slow the Spread." White House, "15 Days to Slow the Spread," March 16, 2020, https://www.whitehouse.gov/articles/15-days-slow-spread.

6. For instance, Jason Mark, "The COVID-19 Rush Never Came to Rural Pennsylvania, and Empty Hospitals Are Feeling the Losses," *Philadelphia Inquirer*, June 16, 2020, https://www.inquirer.com/news/rural-covid-coronavirus-pennsylvania-virus-hospital-health-20200616.html.

7. "Non-Pharmaceutical Public Health Measures for Mitigating the Risk and Impact of Epidemic and Pandemic Influenza," World Health Organization, 2019, https://apps.who.int/iris/bitstream/handle/10665/329438/9789241516839-eng.pdf.

8. Carrie Reed et al., "Novel Framework for Assessing Epidemiologic Effects of Influenza Epidemics and Pandemics," CDC, *Emerging Infectious Diseases* 19, no. 1 (January 2013): 85–91, https://wwwnc.cdc.gov/eid/article/19/1/12-0124_article.

9. "Pandemic Influenza Plan," U.S. Department of Health and Human Services, last updated December 2017, https://www.cdc.gov/flu/pandemic-resources/pdf/pan-flu-report-2017v2.pdf.

10. CDC Director Robert Redfield recommended that several states lock down. Katelyn Caralle, "CDC Director Says He Recommended Some States Lock Down in February as Reports Indicate White House Knew of Coronavirus Threat before They Let on and Donald Trump Retweets '#fireFauci,'" *Daily Mail*, April 13, 2020, https://www.dailymail.co.uk/news/article-8214297/CDC-Director-Robert-Redfield-says-recommended-states-lock-February.html.

11. "Q&A: Influenza and COVID-19—Similarities and Differences," World Health Organization, March 17, 2020, https://www.who.int/emergencies/diseases/novel-coronavirus-2019/question-and-answers-hub/q-a-detail/q-a-similarities-and-differences-covid-19-and-influenza.

12. Timo Smieszek, Gianrocco Lazzari, and Marcel Salathe, "Assessing the Dynamics and Control of Droplet- and Aerosol-Transmitted Influenza Using an Indoor Positioning System," *Nature* 9, no. 2185 (February 2019): 1–10, https://www.nature.com/articles/s41598-019-38825-y.

13. Greg Hudson, "How Often Do You Touch Your Face—and Does That Increase Your Risk for Coronavirus?" *The Hill*, March 2, 2020,

https://thehill.com/changing-america/well-being/
prevention-cures/485519-how-often-do-people-touch-their-face-and-
how-is.

14. Jan Gralton et al., "The Role of Particle Size in Aerosolised Pathogen
Transmission: A Review," *Journal of Infection* 62, no. 1 (January
2011): 1–13, https://www.journalofinfection.com/article/S0163-
4453(10)00347-6/fulltext; William G. Lindsley et al., "Quantity and
Size Distribution of Cough-Generated Aerosol Particles Produced by
Influenza Patients during and after Illness," *Journal of Occupational
and Environmental Hygiene* 9, no. 7 (May 2012): 443–49, https://
www.tandfonline.com/doi/full/10.1080/15459624.2012.684582;
David A. Edwards et al., "Inhaling to Mitigate Exhaled Bioaerosols,"
*Proceedings of the National Academy of Sciences of the United
States*, no. 50 (December 2004), https://www.pnas.org/content/
pnas/101/50/17383.full.pdf.

15. "Valentyn Stadnytskyi et al., "The Airborne Lifetime of Small Speech
Droplets and Their Potential Importance in SARS-CoV-2
Transmission," *Proceedings of the National Academy of Sciences of
the United States* 117, no. 22, (May 13, 2020): 11875–11877, https://
www.pnas.org/content/early/2020/05/12/2006874117.long.

16. "Limiting Spread: Limiting the Spread of Pandemic, Zoonotic, and
Seasonal Epidemic Influenza," World Health Organization, 2010,
https://www.who.int/influenza/resources/research/research_agenda_
influenza_stream_2_limiting_spread.pdf.

17. Smieszek, Lazzari, and Salathe, "Assessing the Dynamics"; Michael P.
Atkinson and Lawrence M. Wein, "Quantifying the Routes of
Transmission for Pandemic Influenza," *Bulletin of Mathematical
Biology* 70 (February 2008): 820–67, https://link.springer.com/article
/10.1007%2Fs11538-007-9281-2; Benjamin J. Cowling et al.,
"Aerosol Transmission Is an Important Mode of Influenza A Virus
Spread," *Nature Communications* 4, no. 1935 (June 2013), https://
www.ncbi.nlm.nih.gov/pmc/articles/PMC3682679; Stadnytskyi et
al., "The Airborne Lifetime of Small Speech Droplets and Their
Potential Importance in SARS-CoV-2 Transmission."

18. Van Doremalen, Bushmaker, and Morris, "Aerosol and Surface
Stability of SARS-CoV-2 as compared with SARS-CoV-1," *The New
England Journal of Medicine*, no. 382 (April 2020): 1564–67, https://
www.nejm.org/doi/full/10.1056/NEJMc2004973.

19. Tze-wai Wong et al., "Cluster of SARS among Medical Students Exposed to Single Patient, Hong Kong," *Emerging Infectious Diseases* 10, no. 2 (February 2004), https://wwwnc.cdc.gov/eid/article/10/2/03-0452-f4.

20. One of the co-authors of this book, William Briggs, was able to observe this in several stores in Taiwan.

21. Nancy Montgomery, "One Meter? Six Feet? How Social Distancing Guidelines Vary across Countries," *Stars & Stripes*, April 7, 2020, https://www.stripes.com/news/europe/one-meter-six-feet-how-social-distancing-guidelines-vary-across-countries-1.625118.

22. Sam Blanchard, "Government Scientific Adviser Says Britain's Two Metre Social Distancing Rule Is Unnecessary and Based on 'Very Fragile' Evidence," *Daily Mail*, May 20, 2020, https://www.dailymail.co.uk/news/article-8339837/Government-scientist-says-2m-social-distancing-rule-based-fragile-evidence.html.

23. Hua Qian et al., "Indoor Transmission of SARS-CoV-2," MedRxiv, April 7, 2020, https://www.medrxiv.org/content/10.1101/2020.04.04.20053058v1.

24. "Non-Pharmaceutical Public Health Measures for Mitigating the Risk and Impact of Epidemic and Pandemic Influenza," World Health Organization, 2019, https://apps.who.int/iris/bitstream/handle/10665/329438/9789241516839-eng.pdf.

25. "Surgeon General Explains Evolution of CDC Face Mask Guidance," MSNBC, April 3, 2020, https://www.msnbc.com/msnbc/watch/surgeon-general-explains-evolution-of-cdc-face-mask-guidance-81619013687.

26. Anna Balazy et al., "Do N95 Respirators Provide 95% Protection Level against Airborne Viruses, and How Adequate Are Surgical Masks?" *American Journal of Infection Control* 34, no. 2 (March 2006): 51–57, https://www.ncbi.nlm.nih.gov/pubmed/16490606.

27. Alyssa Pereira and Brandon Mercer, "Wait, Kids & People with Breathing Problems Should NOT Wear N95 Masks?" *SFGate*, November 16, 2018, https://www.sfgate.com/california-wildfires/article/n95-masks-county-health-safe-advice-doctor-13399569.php.

28. The big unknowns are the prevalence of airborne transmission, the distribution of viral doses in typical airborne transmission events, and the relationship between viral dose and clinical outcome. Speech can produce thousands of virus-containing droplets. Stadnytskyi, Bax,

Bax, and Anfinrud, "The Airborne Lifetime of Small Speech
Droplets." Tests using influenza A to infect ferrets have shown that
ten particles are plenty. John A. Lednicky et al., "Ferrets Develop
Fatal Influenza after Inhaling Small Particle Aerosols of Highly
Pathogenic Avian Influenza Virus A/Vietnam/1203/2004 (H5N1),"
Virology Journal 7, no. 231 (September 2010), https://link.springer.
com/article/10.1186/1743-422X-7-231.

29. Scottie Andrew and James Froio, "These Are the States That Require
You to Wear a Face Mask in Public," CNN, April 20, 2020, https://
www.cnn.com/2020/04/20/us/states-that-require-masks-trnd/index.
html.

30. "Guidance for Cloth Face Coverings," Los Angeles County
Department of Public Health, May 4, 2020, http://publichealth.
lacounty.gov/media/Coronavirus/GuidanceClothFaceCoverings.pdf.

31. Ibid.

Chapter 9: Did the Lockdowns Work?

1. F. A. Hayek, *The Road to Serfdom* (Chicago: University of Chicago
Press, 2007).

2. Katelyn Newman, "Hospital Beds Will Be in Greatest Demand by
Mid-April," U.S. *News and World Report*, March 26, 2020, https://
www.usnews.com/news/best-states/articles/2020-03-26/
us-coronavirus-deaths-hospital-demands-likely-to-hit-peak-in-mid-
april-study.

3. Alan Feuer and Jesse McKinley, "Virus Deaths Mount, but N.Y.
Avoids Predicted Surge at Hospitals So Far," *New York Times*, April
10, 2020, https://www.nytimes.com/2020/04/10/nyregion/new-york-
coronavirus-hospitals.html.

4. NBC News, "White House Coronavirus Briefing," YouTube, April 4,
2020, https://www.youtube.com/
watch?time_continue=66&v=MfxVHK_fr90&feature=emb_logo.

5. Alan Feuer and Jesse McKinley, "Virus Deaths Mount, but N.Y.
Avoids Predicted Surge at Hospitals So Far," *New York Times*, April
10, 2020, https://www.nytimes.com/2020/04/10/nyregion/new-york-
coronavirus-hospitals.html.

6. Richard Sisk, "Underused *Comfort* to Leave NYC, Prepare for
Another Pandemic Mission if Needed," Military.com, April 25, 2020,
https://www.military.com/daily-news/2020/04/25/underused-
comfort-leave-nyc-prepare-another-pandemic-mission-if-needed.html.

7. Carl Campanile and Natalie Musumeci, "$21M Brooklyn Field Hospital Never Saw a Patient amid Coronavirus Pandemic," *New York Post*, May 22, 2020, https://nypost.com/2020/05/22/brooklyn-field-hospital-never-saw-a-coronavirus-patient/.

8. Brandon Specktor, "Coronavirus: What Is 'Flattening the Curve' and Will It Work?" Live Science, March 16, 2020, https://www.livescience.com/coronavirus-flatten-the-curve.html.

9. Jantien A. Backer, Don Klinkenberg, and Jacco Wallinga, "Incubation Period of 2019 Novel Coronavirus (2019-nCoV) Infections among Travellers from Wuhan, China, 20–28 January 2020," *Euro Surveillance* 25, no. 5 (February 2020), https://www.ncbi.nlm.nih.gov/pmc/articles/PMC7014672.

10. "Boris Johnson Announces Police-Enforced Lockdown across the UK to Stop Coronavirus," Heart, March 23, 2020, https://www.heart.co.uk/news/boris-johnson-announces-lockdown.

11. Our World in Data, https://ourworldindata.org.

12. Matt Hancock, "Coronavirus: Matt Hancock Sets Goal of 100,000 Tests Per Day by End of April," *The Guardian*, April 2, 2020, https://www.theguardian.com/politics/video/2020/apr/02/coronavirus-matt-hancock-sets-goal-of-100000-tests-per-day-by-end-of-april-video.

13. "Q&A: Influenza and COVID-19—Similarities and Differences," World Health Organization, March 17, 2020, https://www.who.int/emergencies/diseases/novel-coronavirus-2019/question-and-answers-hub/q-a-detail/q-a-similarities-and-differences-covid-19-and-influenza.

14. "Executive Order N-33-20," Executive Department State of California, March 19, 2020, https://covid19.ca.gov/img/Executive-Order-N-33-20.pdf.

15. Melody Petersen and Emily Baumgaertner, "Bottlenecks in Coronavirus Testing Mean Excruciating Wait Times for the Sick," *Los Angeles Times*, March 30, 2020, https://www.latimes.com/business/story/2020-03-30/its-taking-up-to-eight-days-to-get-coronavirus-tests-results-heres-why.

16. Alex Putterman, "Connecticut Has One of the Nation's Largest COVID-19 Outbreaks but Lags behind Other States in Testing. Here's Why That Is and Why It Matters," *Hartford Courant*, April 6, 2020, https://www.courant.com/coronavirus/

hc-news-coronavirus-covid-19-testing-drive-through-numbers-0402-20200406-yi7fymio3bejfo66i3h2nr4ksq-story.html.

17. David Leonhardt, "How Virus Data Can Mislead: and What Else You Need to Know Today," *New York Times*, May 18, 2020, https://www.nytimes.com/2020/05/18/briefing/coronavirus-world-health-organization-mike-pompeo-monday-briefing.html.

18. Our World in Data, https://ourworldindata.org; "The COVID Tracking Project," The COVID Tracking Project: *The Atlantic*, https://covidtracking.com/api; Sarah Mervosh and Jack Healy, "Holdout States Resist Calls for Stay-at-Home Orders: 'What Are You Waiting For?'" *New York Times*, April 3, 2020, https://www.nytimes.com/interactive/2020/us/coronavirus-stay-at-home-order.html.

19. "COVID-19 Coronavirus Pandemic," Worldometer, last updated July 29, 2020, https://www.worldometers.info/coronavirus.

20. "Philippines Extends Capital's Coronavirus Lockdown to May 15," *Bangkok Post*, April 24, 2020, https://www.bangkokpost.com/world/1906740/philippines-extends-capitals-coronavirus-lockdown-to-may-15.

21. "COVID-19 Coronavirus Pandemic," Worldometer, https://www.worldometers.info/coronavirus.

22. "Coronavirus: Belgium Unveils Plans to Lift Lockdown," BBC News, April 25, 2020, https://www.bbc.com/news/world-europe-52421723.

23. Worldometer, May 13, 2020, https://www.worldometers.info/coronavirus.

24. Entire table is online at https://wmbriggs.com/public/worldometer13may.csv.

25. "Coronavirus Government Response Tracker," University of Oxford, https://www.bsg.ox.ac.uk/research/research-projects/coronavirus-government-response-tracker.

26. Alasdair Sandford, "Coronavirus: Half of Humanity Now on Lockdown as 90 Countries Call for Confinement," Euronews, April 3, 2020, https://www.euronews.com/2020/04/02/coronavirus-in-europe-spain-s-death-toll-hits-10-000-after-record-950-new-deaths-in-24-hou.

27. Vietnam, which reported zero deaths (with lockdown), does not appear (this is a technical limitation because zero doesn't exist on log scales).

28. "Botswana Coronavirus: Govt Prioritizes Data amid Stay Away Campaign," Africa News, May 25, 2020,https://www.africanews.com/2020/05/11/botswana-president-in-self-isolation-after-namibia-trip.

29. "Ethiopia Declares State of Emergency to Fight Coronavirus," Aljazeera, April 8, 2020, https://www.aljazeera.com/news/2020/04/ethiopia-declares-state-emergency-fight-covid-19-200408142519485.html.

30. Abdur Rahman Alfa Shaban, "Ethiopia Coronavirus: Key Updates between March 16-May 16," Africa News, May 19, 2020, https://www.africanews.com/2020/05/10/ethiopia-s-coronavirus-rules-crowd-ban-free-transport-regulate-essentials-etc.

31. Dezan Shira et al., "Vietnam Business Operations and the Coronavirus: Updates," Vietnam Briefing, May 26, 2020, https://www.vietnam-briefing.com/news/vietnam-business-operations-and-the-coronavirus-updates.html.

32. "Deaths Involving COVID-19 by Local Area and Socioeconomic Deprivation: Deaths Occurring between 1 March and 17 April 2020," Office of National Statistics, May 1, 2020, https://www.ons.gov.uk/peoplepopulationandcommunity/birthsdeathsandmarriages/deaths/bulletins/deathsinvolvingcovid19bylocalareasanddeprivation/latest. See also Nathaniel Barker, "The Housing Pandemic: Four Graphs Showing the Link between COVID-19 Deaths and the Housing Crisis," Inside Housing, May 29, 2020, https://www.insidehousing.co.uk/insight/insight/the-housing-pandemic-four-graphs-showing-the-link-between-covid-19-deaths-and-the-housing-crisis-66562. The studies were meant to shed light on over-crowded conditions of some housing, and not to suggest the lockdown exacerbated deaths, but that interpretation is consistent with the data.

33. A possible criticism is that these graphs don't account for population density or other relevant factors including hospital availability, age distribution of the population, mask usage, airline restrictions, and so forth. All true. Population density matters, as in New York City and Los Angeles, which had high death rates. But then again, the densely populated no-lockdown Tokyo, Taipei, and Rio had fewer deaths per capita, so there's more to the story. In any case, we're not trying to explain why deaths varied so much from place to place. We're only showing that they did, colossally, and that there's no proof that the

enormous variation can be explained by the lockdowns. Our point is simple: the data does not show lockdowns work. A criticism that one of us received is that the data (at least the data from some countries) on which we base this argument can't be trusted. There are too many countries, with diverse ways of reporting, different levels of trust in the data and the people reporting that data, suspicious governments, duplicitous media, and so on. Too true! But we can't move from "We have bad data" to "We know lockdowns work based on data." We have to pick one. The coronavirus, as viruses will, found its way to all corners of the world, and it affected different areas differently. That's what the data show. See William M. Briggs, "Bad Arguments for Lockdowns & the Burden of Proof. Also: US States Analysis," WMBriggs.com, May 18, 2020, https://wmbriggs.com/post/30884.

34. There will at least be periodic panics. Right at the end of May came this headline from the *New York Post*: "Scientists Say an Apocalyptic Bird Flu Could Wipe Out Half of Humanity." That the article featured a scientist flogging the book *How to Survive a Pandemic* may have had something to do with it. Paula Froelich, "Scientists Say an Apocalyptic Bird Flu Could Wipe Out Half of Humanity," *New York Post*, May 30, 2020, https://nypost.com/2020/05/30/apocalyptic-bird-flu-could-wipe-out-half-of-humanity-scientists.

35. "Non-Pharmaceutical Public Health Measures for Mitigating the Risk and Impact of Epidemic and Pandemic Influenza," World Health Organization, 2019, https://apps.who.int/iris/bitstream/handle/10665/329438/9789241516839-eng.pdf.

36. Gypsyamber D'Souza and David Dowdy, "What is Herd Immunity and How Can We Achieve It With COVID-19?" Johns Hopkins COVID-19 School of Public Health Expert Insights, April 10, 2020, https://www.jhsph.edu/covid-19/articles/achieving-herd-immunity-with-covid19.html.

37. Noah Higgins-Dunn and Kevin Breuninger, "Cuomo Says It's 'Shocking' Most New Coronavirus Hospitalizations Are People Who Had Been Staying Home," CNBC, May 6, 2020, https://www.cnbc.com/2020/05/06/ny-gov-cuomo-says-its-shocking-most-new-coronavirus-hospitalizations-are-people-staying-home.html.

38. Ibid.

39. Ibid.

CHAPTER 10: THE HUMAN COST

1. Henry David Thoreau, *Walden, or Life in the Woods* (1854).
2. "Flu Costs the U.S. More Than $87 Billion Annually," CDC Foundation, September 18, 2014, https://www.cdcfoundation.org/pr/flu-costs-United-States-87-billion-annually; Kari Paul, "This Year's Flu Season Could Be the Deadliest in Years—and the Most Expensive," Market Watch, February 2, 2018, https://www.marketwatch.com/story/this-is-how-much-this-years-flu-season-could-cost-you-2018-01-09.
3. Geoffrey Joyce, "Opinion: Are We Overreacting to the Coronavirus? Let's Do the Math," Market Watch, April 25, 2020, https://www.marketwatch.com/story/are-we-overreacting-to-the-coronavirus-lets-do-the-math-2020-04-19. Joyce went on to argue that since the lockdown prevented so many more deaths, it was worth it, even if it cost several trillion dollars. But this argument is based on his assumption that policy should respond to the worst-case scenario: "When the virus threat is over, the second-guessing on every policy step and misstep will be cacophonous. But we should remember that when the risk is extreme, such as it is for global warming or COVID-19, public policies should be based on credible worst-case scenarios. Too much is at stake to act otherwise." We discuss this deeply misguided view in chapter 12.
4. Thomas A. Garrett, "Pandemic Economics: The 1918 Influenza and Its Modern-Day Implications," *Federal Reserve Bank of St. Louis Review* 90, no. 2 (March/April 2008): 75–93, https://files.stlouisfed.org/files/htdocs/publications/review/08/03/Garrett.pdf.
5. Thomas A. Garrett, "Economic Effects of the 1918 Influenza Pandemic: Implications for a Modern-day Pandemic," *Federal Reserve Bank of St. Louis* (November 2007): 1–25, https://www.stlouisfed.org/~/media/files/pdfs/community-development/research-reports/pandemic_flu_report.pdf.
6. Sergio Correia, Stephan Luck, and Emil Verner, "Pandemics Depress the Economy, Public Health Interventions Do Not: Evidence from the 1918 Flu," *Social Science Research Network* (March 2020): 1–56, https://papers.ssrn.com/sol3/Papers.cfm?abstract_id=3561560.
7. Pedro Nicolaci da Costa, "Pandemic Economics: Lessons from the Spanish Flu in 1918," *Forbes*, April 3, 2020, https://www.forbes.com/sites/pedrodacosta/2020/04/03/pandemic-economics-lessons-from-the-spanish-flu-in-1918/#5416511b797a; Dylan Matthews, "Social

Distancing Won't Just Save Lives. It Might Be Better for the Economy in the Long Run," Vox, March 31, 2020, https://www.vox.com/future-perfect/2020/3/31/21199874/coronavirus-spanish-flu-social-distancing.

8. Eric Felten, "How Woodrow Wilson Let Flu Deaths Go Viral in the Great War," RealClearInvestigations, April 8, 2020, https://www.realclearinvestigations.com/articles/2020/04/08/how_woodrow_wilson_let_death_run_viral_in_the_great_war_123047.html.

9. Bruce Thompson, "Actual Size of Coronavirus Relief Bill Much Larger Than $2.2 Trillion," Washington Examiner, April 6, 2020, https://www.washingtonexaminer.com/opinion/actual-size-of-coronavirus-relief-bill-much-larger-than-2-2-trillion.

10. Carmen Reinicke, "Credit Suisse Says the US Economy Will Shrink 33.5% Next Quarter, the Biggest Drop in History," Business Insider, April 6, 2020, https://www.businessinsider.com/us-economy-shrink-record-second-quarter-recession-coronavirus-credit-suisse-2020-4.

11. Christos Makridis and Jonathan Hartley, "The Cost of COVID-19: A Rough Estimate of the 2020 US GDP Impact," Mercatus Center, April 6, 2020, https://www.mercatus.org/publications/covid-19-policy-brief-series/cost-covid-19-rough-estimate-2020-us-gdp-impact.

12. By the way, that translates to 6,666,666 life years per month.

13. Sarah Chaney and Gwynn Guilford, "Millions of U.S. Workers Filed for Unemployment Benefits Last Week," Wall Street Journal, April 23, 2020, https://www.wsj.com/articles/millions-of-u-s-workers-continue-to-seek-unemployment-help-amid-coronavirus-11587634201.

14. Jeff Cox, "Another 2.1 million File Jobless Claims, but Total Unemployed Shrinks," CNBC, May 28, 2020, https://www.cnbc.com/2020/05/28/weekly-jobless-claims.html.

15. "Why 1.4 Million Health Jobs Have Been Lost during a Huge Health Crisis," New York Times, 4 May 2020, https://www.nytimes.com/2020/05/08/upshot/health-jobs-plummeting-virus.html.

16. "Employment Situation Summary," U.S. Bureau of Labor Statistics, May 8, 2020, https://www.bls.gov/news.release/empsit.nr0.htm.

17. Peter Coy and Charles Daly, "The Swedish Model Trades More Disease for Less Economic Damage," BloombergQuint, last updated May 18, 2020, https://www.bloombergquint.com/businessweek/sweden-coronavirus-response-less-economic-damage-more-disease.

18. Samantha Chang, "Dan Bongino: My Friend Hanged Himself after Losing His Job Due to Coronavirus Shutdowns," BPR Business & Politics, April 22, 2020, https://www.bizpacreview.com/2020/04/22/dan-bongino-shares-how-a-friend-hung-himself-over-shutdown-in-emotionally-charged-tweet-911595.

19. Nicole Saphier (@NBSaphierMD), "As unemployment approaches 20%, each 1% rise can result in 3.3% spike in drug OD/ 1% increase in suicides (National Bureau of Economic Research.) If unemployment hits 32%, ~77,000 Americans may die as a result. Will economic fallout mortality be greater than the virus itself?" Twitter, April 21, 2020, 1:27 p.m., https://twitter.com/NBSaphierMD/status/1252776683129708545?ref_src=twsrc%5Etfw.

20. Amy Hollyfield, "Suicides on the Rise amid Stay-at-Home Order, Bay Area Medical Professionals Say," ABC7 News, May 21, 2020, https://abc7news.com/suicide-covid-19-coronavirus-rates-during-pandemic-death-by/6201962.

21. Joshua Rhett Miller, "British Teen Dies after Suicide Attempt Due to Coronavirus Fears," *New York Post*, March 25, 2020, https://nypost.com/2020/03/25/british-teen-dies-after-suicide-attempt-due-to-coronavirus-fears/; Tina Moore and Olivia Bensimon, "Man with Cancer Commits Suicide at NYC Hospital after Getting Coronavirus," *New York Post,* March 27, 2020, https://nypost.com/2020/03/27/man-with-cancer-commits-suicide-at-nyc-hospital-after-getting-coronavirus.

22. Kate Briquelet, "Don't Forget the Other Pandemic Killing Thousands of Americans. Authorities Nationwide Are Reporting an Uptick in Fatal Opioid Overdoses during Social Distancing," The Daily Beast, May 4, 2020, https://www.thedailybeast.com/opioid-deaths-surge-during-coronavirus-in-americas-overdose-capitals; TheBlaze (@theblaze), "Nearly three dozen people died in Ontario because coronavirus policies delayed their heart surgeries," Twitter, May 4, 2020, 8:00 p.m., https://twitter.com/theblaze/status/1257505350238044160?s=20; Mallory Simon, "75,000 Americans at Risk of Dying from Overdose or Suicide Due to Coronavirus Despair, Group Warns," CNN, May 8, 2020, https://edition.cnn.com/2020/05/08/health/coronavirus-deaths-of-despair/index.html.

23. Mark A. Reger, Ian H. Stanley, and Thomas E. Joiner, "Suicide Mortality and Coronavirus Disease 2019—a Perfect Storm?" *JAMA Psychiatry*, April 10, 2020, https://jamanetwork.com/journals/jamapsychiatry/fullarticle/2764584.

24. Mayowa Oyesanya, Javier Lopez-Morinigo, and Rina Dutta, "Systematic Review of Suicide in Economic Recession," *World Journal of Psychiatry 5*, no. 2 (June 2015): 243–54, https://www.wjgnet.com/2220-3206/full/v5/i2/243.htm.

25. Eileen Abbott, "How Does the Coronavirus Pandemic Affect Suicide Rates?" *The Hill*, April 22, 2020, https://thehill.com/changing-america/well-being/mental-health/494170-how-does-the-coronavirus-pandemic-affect-suicide.

26. Josh Boswell, "Exclusive: Los Angeles Suicide Hotline Has Received Upwards of 1,500 Calls in March—75 Times the Previous Month—over Fears of Getting Coronavirus and Related Anxiety about Eviction, Inability to Pay Bills and Losing Loved Ones," *Daily Mail*, March 30, 2020, https://www.dailymail.co.uk/news/article-8169429/Los-Angeles-suicide-hotline-received-upwards-1-500-calls-coronavirus-fears.html.

27. Serena Gordon, "Coronavirus Pandemic May Lead to 75,000 'Deaths of Despair' from Suicide, Drug and Alcohol Abuse, Study Says," CBS News, May 8, 2020, https://www.cbsnews.com/news/coronavirus-deaths-suicides-drugs-alcohol-pandemic-75000. The study referred to is Stephen Petterson, John M. Westfall, and Benjamin F. Miller, "Projected Deaths of Despair from COVID-19," Well Being Trust, May 8, 2020, https://wellbeingtrust.org/wp-content/uploads/2020/05/WBT_Deaths-of-Despair_COVID-19-FINAL-FINAL.pdf.

28. Andrew Glen and James Agresti, "Anxiety from Reactions to COVID-19 Will Destroy at Least Seven Times More Years of Life Than Can Be Saved by Lockdowns," The Stream, May 5, 2020, https://stream.org/anxiety-from-reactions-to-covid-19-will-destroy-at-least-seven-times-more-years-of-life-than-can-be-saved-by-lockdowns.

29. Kate Linthicum, Nabih Bulos, and Ana Ionova, "The Economic Devastation Wrought by the Pandemic Could Ultimately Kill More People than the Virus Itself," *Los Angeles Times*, May 11, 2020, https://www.latimes.com/world-nation/story/2020-05-11/

more-than-a-billion-people-escaped-poverty-in-the-last-20-years-the-coronavirus-could-erase-those-gains.

30. Annie Lowrey, "Income Gap, Meet the Longevity Gap," *New York Times,* March 15, 2014, https://www.nytimes.com/2014/03/16/business/income-gap-meet-the-longevity-gap.html.

31. Will Stone and Elly Yu, "Eerie Emptiness of ERs Worries Doctors: Where Are the Heart Attacks and Strokes?" NPR, May 6, 2020, https://www.npr.org/sections/health-shots/2020/05/06/850454989/eerie-emptiness-of-ers-worries-doctors-where-are-the-heart-attacks-and-strokes.

32. Katie Hafner, "Fear of Covid Leads Other Patients to Decline Critical Treatment," *New York Times,* May 25, 2020, https://www.nytimes.com/2020/05/25/health/coronavirus-cancer-heart-treatment.html.

33. Tara Bannow, "Healthcare Loses 1.4 Million Jobs in April as Unemployment Rate Hits 14.7%," Modern Healthcare, May 8, 2020, https://www.modernhealthcare.com/finance/healthcare-loses-14-million-jobs-april-unemployment-rate-hits-147.

34. "35 Cardiac Patients Have Died While Waiting for Surgeries; Ontario to Detail Sector-Specific Reopening Guidelines This week," NOW, April 28, 2020, https://nowtoronto.com/news/april-28-coronavirus-updates-toronto-news.

35. Richard Franki, "Three Months of COVID-19 May Mean 80,000 Missed Cancer Diagnoses," Medscape, May 5, 2020, https://www.medscape.com/viewarticle/929986.

36. Victor Garcia, "Dr. Atlas on Coronavirus Lockdowns: 'The Policy…Is Killing People,'" Fox News, May 24, 2020, https://www.foxnews.com/media/dr-atlas-on-coronavirus-lockdowns-the-policy-is-killing-people.

37. Scott W. Atlas et al., "The COVID-19 Shutdown Will Cost Americans Millions of Years of Life," *The Hill,* May 25, 2020, https://thehill.com/opinion/healthcare/499394-the-covid-19-shutdown-will-cost-americans-millions-of-years-of-life.

38. Aarian Marshall, "Why Farmers Are Dumping Milk, Even as People Go Hungry," *Wired,* April 23, 2020, https://www.wired.com/story/why-farmers-dumping-milk-people-hungry.

39. Tyne Morgan, "Some Growers Plow Under Fields As Fruit, Vegetable Demand Disappears," The Packer, April 20, 2020, https://www.

thepacker.com/article/
some-growers-plow-under-fields-fruit-vegetable-demand-disappears.

40. Christopher Bedford, "How and Why America's Food System is Cracking," The Federalist, May 14, 2020, https://thefederalist. com/2020/05/14/how-and-why-americas-food-system-is-cracking.

41. Mike Hughlett and Adam Belz, "In Minnesota, 10,000 Pigs Are Being Euthanized a Day," Star Tribune, May 6, 2020, https://www. startribune.com/ in-minnesota-10-000-pigs-are-being-euthanized-a-day/570222062.

42. Brad Streicher, "Hundreds Accused of Felony Crimes Released from Travis County Jail," KVUE ABC, April 10, Updated April 11, 2020, https://www.kvue.com/article/news/investigations/defenders/ hundreds-accused-of-felony-crimes-released-from-travis-county-jail/269-8a1bf44d-dcee-426c-8097-c82938a493b1.

43. Ben Johnson, "The Great Coronavirus Jailbreak," The Stream, May 1, 2020, https://stream.org/the-great-coronavirus-jailbreak. A federal judge denied the ACLU request. David Lee, "Judge Won't Release Medically Vulnerable Dallas Jail Inmates," Courthouse News Service, April 27, 2020, https://www.courthousenews.com/ federal-judge-rejects-request-for-release-of-medically-vulnerable-dallas-county-jail-inmates.

44. Craig McCarthy, Ruth Weissmann, and Jorge Fitz-Gibbon, "Dozens of NYC Inmates Back in Jail after Coronavirus Release," New York Post, April 19, 2020, https://nypost.com/2020/04/19/ dozens-of-nyc-inmates-back-in-jail-after-coronavirus-release.

45. Johnson, "The Great Coronavirus Jailbreak."

46. Mike Baker, "Feds Suspect Vast Fraud Network Is Targeting U.S. Unemployment Systems," New York Times, May 16, 2020, https:// www.nytimes.com/2020/05/16/us/coronavirus-unemployment-fraud-secret-service-washington.html.

47. Amber Milne, "'I Had No Choice': Sex for Rent Rises with Coronavirus Poverty," Reuters, May 21, 2020, https://www.reuters. com/article/ us-britain-housing-harassment-trfn/i-had-no-choice-sex-for-rent-rises-with-coronavirus-poverty-idUSKBN22X2N7.

48. Matt Stout, "Reports of Child Abuse and Neglect are Plummeting across New England. That's Not a Good Thing," Boston Globe, April 9, 2020, https://www.bostonglobe.com/2020/04/09/nation/

reports-child-abuse-neglect-are-plummeting-across-new-england-thats-not-good-thing.

49. "More Injured Children Are Visiting ER, Doctor Says," 12 On Your Side, May 15, 2020, https://www.nbc12.com/2020/05/15/more-injured-children-are-visiting-er-doctor-says.

50. "Privacy-Preserving Contact Tracing," Apple, https://www.apple.com/covid19/contacttracing.

51. Sam Biddle, "Coronavirus Monitoring Bracelets Flood the Market, Ready to Snitch on People Who Don't Distance," The Intercept, May 25, 2020, https://theintercept.com/2020/05/25/coronavirus-tracking-bracelets-monitors-surveillance-supercom.

52. Alix Martichoux, "'I Will Not Enforce It': Humboldt Sheriff Says Governor's Beach Closure Would Violate Constitutional Rights," ABC News, April 30, 2020, https://abc7news.com/humboldt-sheriff-beach-newsom-in-california-open/6140197; Tom Tapp, "California Governor Gavin Newsom Closes Orange County Beaches; O.C. Sheriff Says He Won't Enforce the Order," Deadline, April 30, 2020, https://deadline.com/2020/04/california-governor-gavin-newsom-beaches-closed-1202922418.

53. Hayley Peterson, "Walmart Clarifies Its Policy on the Sale of Nonessential Goods after a Shopper Said She Was Barred from Buying a Baby Car Seat," Business Insider, April 13, 2020, https://www.businessinsider.com/walmart-clarifies-policy-on-nonessential-items-after-car-seat-backlash-2020-4.

54. The Hill (@thehill), "Gov. Gretchen Whitmer: "Everything I'm doing is trying to save your life," Twitter, May 15, 2020 6:45 p.m., https://twitter.com/thehill/status/1261427388161744896.

55. R. J. Rummel, Death by Government (New Brunswick: Transaction Publishers, 1994), https://www.hawaii.edu/powerkills/NOTE1.HTM.

56. Samuel Gregg, "The Great Price of America's Great Lockdown," Public Discourse, May 4, 2020, https://www.thepublicdiscourse.com/2020/05/62783.

57. Barnard A. Hebda, Letter to Governor Tim Walz, Archdiocese of Saint Paul and Minneapolis, May 20, 2020, https://s3.amazonaws.com/becketnewsite/Letter-to-Governor-Tim-Walz-May-20-2020-R.pdf.

58. Tyler O'Neil, "Victory for Civil Disobedience: Gov. Loosens Church Restrictions after Catholics, Lutherans Unite," PJ Media, May 23, 2020, https://pjmedia.com/news-and-politics/tyler-o-neil/2020/05/23/minn-gov-loosens-restrictions-on-churches-after-catholics-and-lutherans-defy-his-order-n422825.

59. David Robson, "The Fear of Coronavirus Is Changing Our Psychology," BBC Future, April 1, 2020, https://www.bbc.com/future/article/20200401-covid-19-how-fear-of-coronavirus-is-changing-our-psychology.

60. "Red-Light Moment: Pornography Is Booming during the Covid-19 Lockdowns," *Economist*, May 10, 2020, https://www.economist.com/international/2020/05/10/pornography-is-booming-during-the-covid-19-lockdown; Webinar: Pornography Addiction Rises During COVID-19, Integrative Life Center, April 27, 2020, https://www.integrativelifecenter.com/wellness-blog/pornography-addiction-rises-during-covid-19.

61. Stefanie Valentic, "A Pandemic within a Pandemic," EHS Today, June 18, 2020, https://www.ehstoday.com/health/article/21134240/a-pandemic-within-a-pandemic-substance-abuse-rises-amid-covid.

62. Debbie Koenig, "Quarantine Weight Gain Not A Joking Matter," WebMD, May 21, 2020, https://www.webmd.com/lung/news/20200521/quarantine-weight-gain-not-a-joking-matter.

63. Peter D. Kramer, "Coronavirus: NY Archdiocese Cancels All Funeral Masses, Limits Graveside Services to Priests," Lohud, March 24, 2020, https://www.lohud.com/story/news/coronavirus/2020/03/24/ny-archdiocese-cancels-funeral-masses/2907632001.

64. "Provisional Death Counts for Coronavirus Disease (COVID-19)," CDC.

65. NCHSData19 (4), https://www.cdc.gov/flu/weekly/weeklyarchives2019-2020/data/NCHSData19.csv.

66. "Provisional Death Counts for Coronavirus Disease (COVID-19), CDC, last updated July 30, 2020, https://www.cdc.gov/nchs/nvss/vsrr/covid19/index.htm; United States Population, Worldometer, https://www.worldometers.info/world-population/us-population.

67. Ibid.

68. To explain the dashed line, on July 1, 2020, the CDC estimated there were between twenty and about fifty thousand non-COVID excess

deaths, caused by such things as heart attacks. Excess Deaths Associated With COVID-19, July 1, 2020, https://www.cdc.gov/nchs/nvss/vsrr/covid19/excess_deaths.htm.

69. "Deaths Registered Weekly from 1993 to 2018 by Region, England and Wales," Office for National Statistics, October 16, 2019, https://www.ons.gov.uk/peoplepopulationandcommunity/birthsdeathsandmarriages/deaths/adhocs/10714deathsregisteredweeklyfrom1993to2018byregionenglandandwales; "Deaths Registered Weekly in England and Wales, Provisional," Office for National Statistics, May 2020, https://www.ons.gov.uk/peoplepopulationandcommunity/birthsdeathsandmarriages/deaths/datasets/weeklyprovisionalfiguresondeathsregisteredinenglandandwales.

70. Shaun Griffin, "Covid-19: 'Staggering Number' of Extra Deaths in Community Is Not Explained by Covid-19," *British Medical Journal* (May 2020): 369, https://www.bmj.com/content/369/bmj.m1931.

CHAPTER 11: LIFE, DEATH, AND THE PURSUIT OF HAPPINESS

1. Tim Hains, "Ezekiel Emanuel: U.S. Must Stay Locked Down for 12–18 Months until There's a Vaccine," RealClear Politics, April 7, 2020, https://www.realclearpolitics.com/video/2020/04/07/ezekiel_emanuel_us_must_stay_locked_down_for_12-18_months_until_theres_a_vaccine.html.

2. Marty Johnson, "Fauci: I Don't Think We Should Shake Hands 'Ever Again,'" *The Hill*, April 8, 2020, https://thehill.com/homenews/administration/491917-fauci-i-dont-think-we-should-shake-hands-ever-again.

3. Michael Specter, "How Anthony Fauci Became America's Doctor," *New Yorker*, April 10, 2020, https://www.newyorker.com/magazine/2020/04/20/how-anthony-fauci-became-americas-doctor.

4. Kevin Freking and Jill Colvin, "Trump Takes Aim at Fauci over Opening Schools in the Fall," *Time*, May 14, 2020, https://time.com/5836648/donald-trump-schools-reopening-anthony-fauci; Jill Filipovic, "Fauci Warns of Colossal Deadly Mistake. Will Trump Listen?" CNN, May 12, 2020, https://www.cnn.com/2020/05/12/opinions/fauci-testimony-trump-administration-response-filipovic/index.html; Lauran Neergaard and Ricardo Alonso-Zaldivar, "Fauci

Warns: More Death, Econ Damage if US Reopens Too Fast," AP News, May 12, 2020, https://apnews.com/e64f20bbacb7d48d15e1d76339220486.

5. Steve Deace, "This is for those in the Cult of Fauci...," LinkedIn, May 14, 2020, https://www.linkedin.com/feed/update/urn:li:activ ity:6666675265621557248.

6. "Potential Years of Life Lost," OECD, https://data.oecd.org/healthstat/potential-years-of-life-lost.htm#indicator-chart.

7. Ibid.

8. Philosopher Robert Koons does an admirable job of analyzing the moral complexities in Robert C. Koons, "Can We Measure the Value of Saving Human Lives in Dollars? Somber Calculations in a Time of Plague," Public Discourse, March 31, 2020, https://www.thepublicdiscourse.com/2020/03/61900.

9. "Weekly Updates by Select Demographic and Geographic Characteristics: Provisional Death Counts for Coronavirus Disease (COVID-19), CDC, https://www.cdc.gov/nchs/nvss/vsrr/covid_weekly/index.htm#AgeAndSex.

10. Kenneth D. Kochanek et al., "Deaths: Final Data for 2017," *National Vital Statistics Reports* 68, no. 9 (June 2019): 1–77, https://www.cdc.gov/nchs/data/nvsr/nvsr68/nvsr68_09-508.pdf.

11. Christopher Davis et al., "Safety is Third, Not First, and We All Know It Should Be," *Journal of Emergency Medical Services*, November 13, 2018, https://www.jems.com/2018/11/13/safety-is-third-not-first-and-we-all-know-it-should-be.

12. Tessa Weinberg, "'More Important Things Than Living,' Texas' Dan Patrick Says in Coronavirus Interview," *Star Telegram*, April 21, 2020, https://www.star-telegram.com/news/politics-government/article242167741.html.

13. See James Broughel and Michael Kotrous, "Why Economists Measure Human Lives in Dollars," *Politico*, April 2, 2020, https://www.politico.com/news/magazine/2020/04/02/coronavirus-economy-reopen-deaths-balance-analysis-159248#1.

14. Vance Ginn, "We Must Learn from the Shutdown Mistake," *The Hill*, June 13, 2020, https://thehill.com/opinion/finance/502518-we-must-learn-from-the-shutdown-mistake.

Chapter 12: Through a Glass Darkly: Balancing Costs with Benefits When We Don't Know the Future

1. Quoted in Larry Prather and Dan Delich, "In Flood Resilience Debate, There Are No Solutions—Only Tradeoffs," *The Hill*, February 2, 2019, https://thehill.com/opinion/energy-environment/428193-in-flood-resilience-debate-there-are-no-solutions-only-tradeoffs.

2. William Feuer, "Fauci Says It's Still Possible That a Coronavirus Vaccine Will Be Available in the U.S. by December," CNBC, May 22, 2020, https://www.cnbc.com/2020/05/22/dr-fauci-is-still-confident-us-could-have-a-coronavirus-vaccine-by-december.html.

3. Daniel Burke, "The Dangerous Morality behind the "Open it Up' Movement," CNN, April 23, 2020, https://www.cnn.com/2020/04/23/us/reopening-country-coronavirus-utilitarianism/index.html.

4. "Restraint Use on Aircraft," *Pediatrics* 108, no. 5 (November 2001): 1218–22, https://pediatrics.aappublications.org/content/108/5/1218.

5. "Fatality Facts 2018 Yearly Snapshot," IIHS, https://www.iihs.org/topics/fatality-statistics/detail/yearly-snapshot; "List of Accidents and Incidents involving Commercial Aircraft," Wikipedia, https://en.wikipedia.org/wiki/List_of_accidents_and_incidents_involving_commercial_aircraft#2004.

6. "Restraint Use on Aircraft," *Pediatrics*.

7. Frédéric Bastiat, "What Is Seen and What is Not Seen" (1950), https://tinyurl.com/y8k36c78.

8. H. Rashid et al., "Evidence Compendium and Advice on Social Distancing and Other Related Measures for Response to an Influenza Pandemic," *Paediatric Respiratory Reviews* 16, no. 2 (March 2015): 119–26, https://pubmed.ncbi.nlm.nih.gov/24630149.

9. Keith McShea, "Human Lives Come First as N.Y. Weighs Reopening, Cuomo Reiterates," *Buffalo News*, May 5, 2020, https://buffalonews.com/2020/05/05/cuomo-says-real-reopening-discussion-is-how-much-is-a-human-life-worth.

10. Anne Case and Angus Deaton, *Deaths of Despair and the Future of Capitalism* (Princeton: Princeton University Press, 2020).

11. There was a drop in total traffic fatalities, but an increase in deaths per mile driven because of more speeding on empty roads. "Motor Vehicle Fatality Rates Up 14 Percent in March, Despite COVID-19," *Occupational Health & Safety*, May 22, 2020, https://ohsonline.com/articles/2020/05/22/motor-vehicle-fatality-rates-up-14-percent-in-march-despite-covid19.aspx.

12. Nassim Nicholas Taleb (@nntaleb), "Another ignorant journalist dealing with risk matters. Irresponsible," Twitter, January 26, 2020, 3:31 p.m., https://twitter.com/nntaleb/status/1221531095864348672.

13. Joseph Norman et al., "Systemic Risk of Pandemic via Novel Pathogens—Coronavirus: A Note," Academia, January 26, 2020, https://www.academia.edu/41743064/Systemic_Risk_of_Pandemic_via_Novel_Pathogens_-_Coronavirus_A_Note.

14. Michael Shermer, "Rumsfeld's Wisdom: Where the Known Meets the Unknown Is Where Science Begins," *Scientific American*, September 1, 2005, https://www.scientificamerican.com/article/rumsfelds-wisdom.

15. "Wingspread Conference on the Precautionary Principle," Wikipedia, https://en.wikipedia.org/wiki/Wingspread_Conference_on_the_Precautionary_Principle.

16. See, for example, Aria Bendix, "Health Experts Issued an Ominous Warning about a Coronavirus Pandemic 3 Months Ago. The Virus in Their simulation Killed 65 Million People," *Business Insider*, January 23, 2020, https://www.businessinsider.com/scientist-simulated-coronavirus-pandemic-deaths-2020-1; John Koetsier, "AI Predicts Coronavirus Could Infect 2.5 Billion and Kill 53 Million. Doctors Say That's Not Credible, and Here's Why," *Forbes*, February 5, 2020, https://www.forbes.com/sites/johnkoetsier/2020/02/05/ai-predicts-coronavirus-could-infect-25b-and-kill-53m-doctors-say-thats-not-credible-and-heres-why/#15a43c5e11cd; Patrick Knox, "Apocalypse Now. Bill Gates 'Predicted' How Coronavirus-Like Pandemic Could Spread Saying 33 MILLION May Die in First Six Months," *U.S. Sun*, January 24, 2020, https://www.the-sun.com/news/306110/bill-gates-predicted-chinese-coronavirus-a-year-ago-as-simulation-suggests-65-million-could-die; Fabienne Lang, "An 'IT Person' Predicted How Many Deaths the Coronavirus Will Really Cause," Interesting Engineering, February 4, 2020, https://interestingengineering.com/

an-it-person-predicted-how-many-deaths-the-coronavirus-will-really-cause; Michael Le Page and Debora Mackenzie, "Could the New Coronavirus Really Kill 50 Million People Worldwide?" *New Scientist*, February 11, 2020, https://www.newscientist.com/article/2233085-could-the-new-coronavirus-really-kill-50-million-people-worldwide.

17. Nassim Nicholas Taleb and Joseph Norman, "Ethics of Precaution: Individual and Systemic Risk," Academia, March 15, 2020, https://www.academia.edu/42223846/Ethics_of_Precaution_Individual_and_Systemic_Risk.

CHAPTER 13: WHO GOT IT RIGHT?

1. "New Coronary Pneumonia Taiwan Outbreak Data," Infogram, https://infogram.com/—h8j4xgy7x1d6mv; Chen Yi'an, "Why Did the 1738 Aquarius Star Check Only 128 people? Scholars Praised the Logic of Epidemic Prevention Staff as 'Smart,'" *Storm*, February 10, 2020, https://www.storm.mg/article/2275639.

2. Sophia Yang, "8 Taiwanese Universities Delay Opening to Stop Coronavirus Spread," *Taiwan News*, February 3, 2020, https://www.taiwannews.com.tw/en/news/3869701.

3. "Guidelines for Large-Scale Public Gatherings in the Wake of the COVID-19 Outbreak (Update: 2020/03/05)," *Ministry of Foreign Affairs Republic of China (Taiwan)*, https://www.mofa.gov.tw/en/cp.aspx?n=5A2D9F78CE42DD4A.

4. Matthew Strong, "Catholic Churches for Filipinos in Taiwan Close over Coronavirus," *Taiwan News*, February 29, 2020, https://www.taiwannews.com.tw/en/news/3883273.

5. Joy Y. T. Chang, "Taiwan Reopens Baseball Stadiums to Fans," SCMP, May 8, 2020, https://www.scmp.com/video/coronavirus/3083616/taiwan-baseball-league-reopens-stadiums-fans.

6. "Entry Restrictions for Foreigners to Taiwan in Response to COVID-19 Outbreak," Bureau of Consular Affairs, Ministry of Foreign Affairs, Republic of China (Taiwan), May 18, 2020, https://www.boca.gov.tw/cp-220-5081-c06dc-2.html.

7. Ibid.

8. "FAQ: Taiwan's 14-Day Quarantine Requirements," *Taiwan Today*, March 18, 2020, https://taiwantoday.tw/news.php?unit=2,6,10,15,18&post=173589.

9. "Entry Restrictions for Foreigners to Taiwan," Bureau of Consular Affairs.

10. "CECC Urges People to Conduct a 14-Day Period of Self-Health Management If They Visit Crowded Places during the Tomb Sweeping Festival," *Taiwan Centers for Disease Control*, April 6, 2020, https://www.cdc.gov.tw/En/Bulletin/Detail/8QT-pWlYfLRq_nBPB7adog?typeid=158.

11. Ying-Hen Hsieh et al., "Quarantine for SARS, Taiwan," *Emerging Infectious Diseases* 11, no. 2 (February 2005): 278-282, https://www.ncbi.nlm.nih.gov/pmc/articles/PMC3320446.

12. Matthew Strong, "Wearing a Face Mask to Become Compulsory on the Taipei MRT from April 4," *Taiwan News*, April 3, 2020, https://www.taiwannews.com.tw/en/news/3909701.

13. Tsai Peng-min and Frances Huang, "Taipei 101, SOGO Say No to Visitors with High Temperatures," *Focus Taiwan*, February 28, 2020, https://focustaiwan.tw/society/202002280013.

14. Mark Moore, "Taiwan Accuses WHO of Downplaying Coronavirus Toll in China," *New York Post*, April 14, 2020, https://nypost.com/2020/04/14/taiwan-accuses-who-of-downplaying-china-coronavirus-spread-reports.

15. Keoni Everington, "WHO Head Accuses Taiwan of Racist Attack, Blames MOFA," *Taiwan News*, April 9, 2020, https://www.taiwannews.com.tw/en/news/3912961.

16. Ching-Tse Cheng, "WHO Chief Blames Taiwan for Soiled Reputation amid Coronavirus Failings," *Taiwan News*, March 27, 2020, https://www.taiwannews.com.tw/en/news/3905515.

17. Keoni Everington, "Tedros Doubles Down on Denial of Taiwan warning," *Taiwan News*, April 21, 2020, https://www.taiwannews.com.tw/en/news/3919947.

18. Marta Paterlini, "'Closing Borders Is Ridiculous': The Epidemiologist behind Sweden's Controversial Coronavirus Strategy," *Nature*, April 21, 2020, https://www.nature.com/articles/d41586-020-01098-x.

19. "Public Health Authorities Have Failed—Now Politicians Must Intervene," DN Debate, April 24, 2020, https://www.dn.se/debatt/folkhalsomyndigheten-har-misslyckats-nu-maste-politikerna-gripa-in.

20. Derek Robertson, "'They Are Leading Us to Catastrophe': Sweden's Coronavirus Stoicism Begins to Jar," *Guardian*, March 30, 2020,

https://www.theguardian.com/world/2020/mar/30/
catastrophe-sweden-coronavirus-stoicism-lockdown-europe.

21. Anders Tegnell, "Sweden's Strategy Is Largely Working—Chief
Epidemiologist," BBC News, April 24, 2020, https://www.bbc.com/
news/av/world-europe-52409414/
sweden-s-strategy-is-largely-working-chief-epidemiologist.

22. Karen Yourish et al., "One-Third of All U.S. Coronavirus Deaths Are
Nursing Home Residents or Workers," *New York Times*, May 11,
2020, https://www.nytimes.com/interactive/2020/05/09/us/
coronavirus-cases-nursing-homes-us.html; Caroline Hurley, "Nursing
Homes Account for More than Half of Coronavirus Deaths in
Illinois, New Data Shows," *Chicago Sun Times*, May 29, 2020,
https://chicago.suntimes.com/coronavirus/2020/5/29/21275284/
nursing-homes-coronavirus-deaths-illinois-data; "Coronavirus: 51%
of COVID-19 Deaths in LA County Were Residents in 'Institutional
Settings,'" ABC7, May 14, 2020, https://abc7.com/
health/5125-of-all-covid-19-deaths-in-la-county-were-residents-in-
institutional-settings/6183073.

23. Sinéad Baker, "The Architect of Sweden's Decision Not to Have a
Coronavirus Lockdown Says He Still Isn't Sure It Was the Right Call,"
Business Insider, May 4, 2020, https://www.businessinsider.com/
coronavirus-sweden-no-lockdown-anders-tegnell-not-convinced-right-
call-2020-5.

24. Epsilon (@epsilon3141), "Sweden has now the highest #covid19
fatality rate per million population of the world. A direct consequence
of the inhumane "herd immunity" plan. Swedens daily #covid19
deaths per million are 100x as many as deaths from traffic accidents
and homicide together," Twitter, May 16, 2020, 6:37 p.m., https://
twitter.com/epsilon3141/status/1261787762107322369.

25. Richard Orange, "Sweden Becomes Country with Highest
Coronavirus Death Rate per Capita over Past Seven Days,"
Telegraph, May 20, 2020, https://www.telegraph.co.uk/
news/2020/05/20/
sweden-becomes-country-highest-coronavirus-death-rate-per-capita.

26. "Norway 'Could Have Controlled Infection without Lockdown':
Health Chief," The Local, May 22, 2020, https://www.thelocal.
no/20200522/
norway-could-have-controlled-infection-without-lockdown-health-
chief.

27. William Sposato, "Japan's Halfhearted Coronavirus Measures Are Working Anyway," *Foreign Policy*, May 14, 2020, https://foreignpolicy.com/2020/05/14/japan-coronavirus-pandemic-lockdown-testing.

28. Jason Lemon, "Japan Ends Coronavirus Emergency With 850 Deaths and No Lockdown," *Newsweek*, May 25, 2020, https://www.newsweek.com/japan-ends-coronavirus-emergency-850-deaths-no-lockdown-1506336.

29. Rupert Wingfield-Hayes, "Coronavirus: Japan's Low Testing Rate Raises Questions," BBC News, April 30, 2020, https://www.bbc.com/news/world-asia-52466834.

30. Tom Feiling, "How Japan's Refusal to Impose a Coronavirus Lockdown Is Dividing the Country," *New Statesman,* April 23, 2020, https://www.newstatesman.com/world/asia/2020/04/japan-lockdown-coronavirus-covid-shinzo-abe.

31. "Japan Rejected Lockdown Because Virus Will Resurge, Says Expert," *Financial Times*, https://www.ft.com/content/9bac4ad5-22e3-4bcd-b07b-8a248fe44465.

32. Riyaz ul Khaliq, "'COVID-19 Did Not Change Much in Japan's Daily Life,'" Anadolu Agency, April 26, 2020, https://www.aa.com.tr/en/asia-pacific/-covid-19-did-not-change-much-in-japan-s-daily-life-/1819015.

33. Gavin Blair, "Japan Suicides Decline as Covid-19 Lockdown Causes Shift in Stress Factors," *Guardian*, May 14, 2020, https://www.theguardian.com/world/2020/may/14/japan-suicides-fall-sharply-as-covid-19-lockdown-causes-shift-in-stress-factors.

34. Dennis Normile, "Japan Ends Its COVID-19 State of Emergency," *Science*, May 26, 2020, https://www.sciencemag.org/news/2020/05/japan-ends-its-covid-19-state-emergency.

35. Holly Secon, "An Interactive Map of the US Cities and States Still under Lockdown—and Those That Are Reopening," *Business Insider*, May 19, 2020, https://www.businessinsider.com/us-map-stay-at-home-orders-lockdowns-2020-3.

36. "US Historical Data," The COVID Tracking Project at *The Atlantic*, https://covidtracking.com/data/us-daily.

37. "Models Project Sharp Rise in Deaths as States Reopen," *New York Times*, last updated May 15, 2020, https://www.nytimes.com/2020/05/04/us/coronavirus-live-updates.html.

38. Lateshia Beachum et al, "Fauci Warns That 'Consequences Could Be Really Serious' if States Move Too Quickly to Reopen," *Washington Post*, May 12, 2020, https://www.washingtonpost.com/nation/2020/05/12/coronavirus-update-us.

39. WTVC, Associated Press, "Kemp: Some Georgia Businesses Allowed to Reopen April 24; Shelter-in-Place to End April 30," ABC News Channel 9, April 20, 2020, https://newschannel9.com/news/local/gov-kemp-certain-georgia-businesses-allowed-to-reopen-april-24.

40. Dana Milbank, "Georgia Leads the Ace to Become America's No. 1 Death Destination," *Washington Post*, April 21, 2020, https://www.washingtonpost.com/opinions/2020/04/21/georgia-leads-race-become-americas-no-1-death-destination.

41. Alexandra Sternlicht, "Georgia Coronavirus Deaths Surpass 1,000; Forecaster Says Will Double by August With Reopening," *Forbes*, April 29, 2020, https://www.forbes.com/sites/alexandrasternlicht/2020/04/29/georgia-coronavirus-deaths-surpass-1000-forecaster-says-will-double-by-august-with-reopening/#3f7c58e43531.

42. Jacqueline Howard, "Georgia's Daily Coronavirus Deaths Will Nearly Double by August with Relaxed Social Distancing, Model Suggests," CNN, April 28, 2020, https://edition.cnn.com/2020/04/28/health/georgia-coronavirus-death-projections/index.html.

43. The COVID Tracking Project shows the seven-day average of new COVID-19 deaths in Georgia going from about forty per day in late April to under twenty per day in early July, with ups and downs in that range along the way. See "Georgia," The COVID Tracking Project at *The Atlantic*, https://covidtracking.com/data/state/georgia.

CHAPTER 14: LESSONS LEARNED

1. Chuck Palahniuk, *Lullaby* (New York: Anchor, 2002), 21.

2. Avik Roy, "The Most Important Coronavirus Statistic: 42% of U.S. Deaths Are from 0.6% of the Population," *Forbes*, May 26, 2020, https://www.forbes.com/sites/theapothecary/2020/05/26/nursing-homes-assisted-living-facilities-0-6-of-the-u-s-population-43-of-u-s-covid-19-deaths/#7a995a5f74cd.

3. Bernadette Hogan and Bruce Golding, "Nursing Homes Have 'No Right' to Reject Coronavirus Patients, Cuomo Says," *New York Post*, April 23, 2020, https://nypost.com/2020/04/23/nursing-homes-cant-reject-coronavirus-patients-cuomo-says.

4. Betsy McCaughey, "New York's Nursing Home Horrors Are Even Worse Than You Think," *New York Post*, May 29, 2020, https://nypost.com/2020/05/29/new-yorks-nursing-home-horrors-are-even-worse-than-you-think; Rich Lowry, "Where Does Ron DeSantis Go to Get His Apology?" *National Review*, May 20, 2020, https://www.nationalreview.com/2020/05/coronavirus-crisis-ron-desantis-florida-covid-19-strategy.

5. Gregg Girvan and Avik Roy, "Nursing Homes & Assisted Living Facilities Account for 42% of COVID-19 Deaths," FREOPP, May 22, 2020, https://freopp.org/the-covid-19-nursing-home-crisis-by-the-numbers-3a47433c3f70.

6. Christine Sexton, "As Coronavirus Cases Rise, Gov. Ron DeSantis Bans Visitors to All Florida Nursing Homes," *Orlando Weekly*, March 15, 2020, https://www.orlandoweekly.com/Blogs/archives/2020/03/15/as-coronavirus-cases-rise-gov-ron-desantis-bans-visitors-to-all-florida-nursing-homes.

7. Stefania Boccia, Walter Ricciardi, and John P. A. Ioannidis, "Evidence from Italy and Elsewhere Suggests that Many Infections Are 'Nosocomial,' That Is, Originating and Spread in Hospitals," *Journal of the American Medical Association* (April 7, 2020), https://jamanetwork.com/journals/jamainternalmedicine/fullarticle/2764369.

8. Rich Lowry, "Where Does Ron DeSantis Go to Get His Apology?"

9. Douglass Dowty, "Cuomo: NY Coronavirus Projections 'All Wrong,' Too Early to Tell if Reopening Is Working," Syracuse.com, May 25, 2020, https://www.syracuse.com/news/2020/05/cuomo-ny-coronavirus-projections-all-wrong-too-early-to-tell-if-reopening-is-working.html.

10. In May 2020 a group of Brazilian experts pointed out that it was "clear that the intention" of authorities claiming all their decisions were based on science was "to lead all of us to the idea of decisions based on something unquestionable and infallible, as scientific as law, as the law of gravity." See "Brazilian Scientists and Academics Write an Open Letter on the 'Science' of the Coronavirus Pandemic,"

Conexao Politica, May 25, 2020, https://conexaopolitica.com.br/
ultimas/
brazilian-scientists-and-academics-write-an-open-letter-on-the-
science-of-the-coronavirus-pandemic.

11. See Roger Koppl, "Pandemics and the Problem of Expert Failure,"
    The Library of Economics and Liberty, March 30, 2020, https://
    www.econlib.org/pandemics-and-the-problem-of-expert-failure.

12. For an extended treatment of the "vocation" of politics, see Bruce K.
    Chapman, *Politicians: The Worst Kind of People to Run the
    Government, Except for All the Others* (Seattle: Discovery Institute
    Press, 2018).

13. The most mature form of Hayek's argument is in *The Fatal Conceit:
    The Errors of Socialism* (Chicago: University of Chicago Press, 1989).

14. Clare Malone and Kyle Bourassa, "Americans Didn't Wait for Their
    Governors to Tell Them to Stay Home Because of COVID-19,"
    FiveThirtyEight, May 8, 2020, https://fivethirtyeight.com/features/
    americans-didnt-wait-for-their-governors-to-tell-them-to-stay-home-
    because-of-covid-19.

15. "An Incalculable Loss," *New York Times*, May 24, 2020, https://
    www.nytimes.com/interactive/2020/05/24/us/us-coronavirus-
    deaths-100000.html?action=click&module=Spotlight&pgtype=Hom
    epage.

16. Justin Hart (@justin_hart), "6th name on the original NYTimes list...
    was actually murdered. The SIXTH name. I expect we'll see some
    more corrections," Twitter, May 24, 2020, 8:13 a.m., https://twitter.
    com/justin_hart/status/1264529912024592384; Bob James, "Man
    Found in Vehicle Along I-380 was Murdered," KHAK, March 20,
    2020, https://khak.com/
    body-found-in-vehicle-near-i-380-cedar-rapids.

17. Joe Nocera, "Lockdowns Haven't Proved They're Worth the Havoc,"
    Bloomberg, May 21, 2020, https://www.bloomberg.com/opinion/
    articles/2020-05-21/
    coronavirus-lockdowns-haven-t-proved-they-re-worth-the-havoc.

18. See, for example, Selena Simmons-Duffin and Nurith Aizenman,
    "Are U.S. Hospitals Ready?" NPR, March 17, 2020, https://www.
    npr.org/sections/health-shots/2020/03/17/815484566/
    are-u-s-hospitals-ready.

19. See, for example, Kanny Malone and Karen Duffin, "The Race to
    Make Ventilators," NPR, March 31, 2020, https://www.npr.

org/2020/03/31/824886286/
episode-987-the-race-to-make-ventilators.

20. See, for example, Noel King, "Snorkel Kits Help Doctors Get through PPE Shortage," NPR, April 23, 2020, https://www.npr. org/2020/04/23/842195578/ snorkel-kits-help-doctors-get-through-ppe-shortage.

21. See, for example, Sacha Pfeiffer, Meg Anderson, and Barbara van Woerkom, "Despite Early Warnings, U.S. Took Months to Expand Swab Production for COVID-19 Test," NPR, May 12, 2020, https:// www.npr.org/2020/05/12/853930147/ despite-early-warnings-u-s-took-months-to-expand-swab-production-for-covid-19-te.

22. Sy Becker, "Holyoke Medical Center Scales Back on Covid-19 Testing Services," WLLP 22 NEWS, June 26, 2020, https://www.wwlp.com/ news/local-news/hampden-county/ holyoke-medical-center-scales-back-on-covid-19-testing-services.

23. See, for example, Morgan Chalfant, "Trump: 'With Smaller Testing We Would Show Fewer Cases,'" *The Hill*, June 23, 2020, https:// thehill.com/homenews/administration/504026-trump-with-smaller-testing-we-would-show-fewer-cases; and Eli Stokols and Janet Hook, "New Coronavirus Spike Alarms Republicans, but Not Trump," *Los Angeles Times*, June 25, 2020, https://www.latimes.com/politics/ story/2020-06-25/ new-coronavirus-spike-alarms-republicans-but-not-trump.

Conclusion: Against the Brave New Normal

1. C. S. Lewis "The Humanitarian Theory of Punishment," *God in the Dock* (Grand Rapids: Eerdmans, 2014), 318–33.

2. Arianna Poindexter, "Mississippi Church Destroyed by Arson Was Suing City over Safer-at-Home Order," WLBT3, May 20, 2020, https://www.wlbt.com/2020/05/20/ mississippi-church-destroyed-by-arson-was-suing-city-holly-springs-over-safer-at-home-order.

3. "Whitmer: Coronavirus Orders Are 'Not Suggestions, Not Optional,'" ABC 12, May 11, 2000, https://www.abc12.com/ content/news/Whitmer-Coronavirus-orders-are-not-suggestions-not-optional-570380331.html.

4. Ariel Zilber, "Michigan Gov. Whitmer Is Accused of Lockdown Hypocrisy after Her 'Husband Tried to Ready Their Boat for Memorial Weekend' 150 Miles from the State Capital—After She Told the Public Not to Travel There," *Daily Mail*, May 25, 2020, https://www.dailymail.co.uk/news/article-8356193/Gretchen-Whitmers-husband-asked-dock-company-boat-water-vacation-home.html.

5. See Ryan Saavedra, "Emails Show Democrat Gretchen Whitmer's Office Gave 'Green Light' to Give Taxpayer Money to Democrat Groups for Contact Tracing, Report Says," Daily Wire, May 26, 2020,https://www.dailywire.com/news/breaking-emails-show-democrat-gretchen-whitmers-office-gave-green-light-to-give-taxpayer-money-to-democrat-groups-for-contact-tracing-report-says.

6. Matt Viser and Josh Dawsey, "Michigan Cancels Contract with Two Democratic-Linked Firms That Had Been Tapped to Track Coronavirus," *Washington Post,* April 21, 2020, https://www.washingtonpost.com/politics/michigan-cancels-contract-with-two-democratic-linked-firms-that-had-been-tapped-to-track-coronavirus/2020/04/21/161a23ce-8413-11ea-ae26-989cfce1c7c7_story.html.

7. David Krayden, "Lockdowns Are Feeding Authoritarian Appetites," *Human Events*, May 29, 2020 https://humanevents.com/2020/05/29/lockdowns-are-feeding-authoritarian-appetites.

8. Ben Yakas, "Video: Brooklyn Politicians Break Open Playgrounds in Defiance of De Blasio," Gothamist, June 16, 2020, https://gothamist.com/news/videos-brooklyn-politicians-break-open-playgrounds-defiance-de-blasio.

9. Matt Zapotosky and Isaac Stanley-Becker, "Gripped by Disease, Unemployment and Outrage at the Police, America Plunges into Crisis," *Washington Post*, May 29, 2020, https://www.washingtonpost.com/national-security/plagued-by-disease-unemployment-and-outrage-at-the-police-america-plunges-into-crisis/2020/05/29/c8329bb2-a1b5-11ea-81bb-c2f70f01034b_story.html; Noah Rothman, "The Riots and the Lockdown," *Commentary*, May 31, 2020, https://www.commentarymagazine.com/noah-rothman/the-riots-and-the-lockdown.

10. Swordfishtrombone (@TheyCallMeRyols), "Replying to @Heminator and @ggreenwald," Twitter, June 14, 2020, 11:03 p.m., https://twitter.com/TheyCallMeRyols/status/1272364102933856256. *Time* had run the first story on June 10. Jamie Ducharme, "'Protest Is a Profound Public Health Intervention': Why So Many Doctors Are Supporting Protests in the Middle of the COVID-19 Pandemic," *Time*, June 10, 2020, https://time.com/5848212/doctors-supporting-protests.

11. Arno Pedram and Sylvia Hui, "Hundreds of Far-Right Protesters Defy COVID-19 Restrictions to Demonstrate in London," *Time*, June 13, 2020, https://time.com/5853234/far-right-protesters-statues-london.

12. Mark Hemingway, "Little over an hour apart," Twitter, Jun 14, 2020, 10:32 p.m., https://twitter.com/Heminator/status/1272356179403059207.

13. Alex vanNess, Twitter, June 22, 2020,1:25 p.m., https://twitter.com/thealexvanness/status/1275117632488955908.

14. Tobias Hoonhout, "Dem Rep. Told Colleagues Coronavirus Bill Is 'Tremendous Opportunity to Restructure Things to Fit Our Vision,'" *National Review*, March 23, 2020, https://www.nationalreview.com/news/dem-rep-told-colleagues-coronavirus-bill-is-tremendous-opportunity-to-restructure-things-to-fit-our-vision.

15. "The HEROES Act: Disturbing Finds in the Dems' New $3 Trillion Relief Bill," The Stream, May 13, 2020, https://stream.org/the-heroes-act-disturbing-finds-in-the-dems-new-3-trillion-relief-bill.

16. See Jonah Goldberg, *Liberal Fascism* (New York: Crown Forum, 2009).

17. Gillian Flaccus and Andrew Selsky, "Oregon Supreme Court Halts Order Nixing Virus Restrictions," AP News, May 18, 2020, https://apnews.com/858075236a56cad769c96c0187b8bfe6.

18. Sarah Mervosh et al., "See Which States and Cities Have Told Residents to Stay at Home," *New York Times*, April 20, 2020, https://www.nytimes.com/interactive/2020/us/coronavirus-stay-at-home-order.html.

19. "Roadmap for the Implementation of Actions by the European Commission Based on the Commission Communication and the Council Recommendation on Strengthening Cooperation against Vaccine Preventable Diseases," European Commission, https://

ec.europa.eu/health/sites/health/files/vaccination/docs/2019-2022_roadmap_en.pdf.

20. "The Great Reset: A Unique Twin Summit to Begin 2021," World Economic Forum, n.d., https://www.weforum.org/great-reset/about.

21. This still might happen, if the Europeans let them get away with it. See Henry T. Greely, "Covid-19 'Immunity Certificates': Practical and Ethical Conundrums," STAT News, April 10, 2020, https://www.statnews.com/2020/04/10/immunity-certificates-covid-19-practical-ethical-conundrums.

22. Tristan Harris, "Silicon Valley, It's Your Chance to Turn the Tide on Covid-19," *Wired*, March 24, 2020, https://www.wired.com/story/opinion-this-is-silicon-valleys-chance-to-step-up-for-humanity.

23. Tina Moore, Gabrielle Fonrouge, and Bruce Golding, "DeBlasio's Social Distancing Tip Line Flooded with Penis Photos, Hitler Memes," *New York Post*, April 21, 2020, https://nypost.com/2020/04/21/de-blasios-social-distancing-tip-line-flooded-with-obscenities.

24. Bruce Haring, "Los Angeles County Residents Ignore 'No Fireworks' Order, Celebrate with Massive Display," Deadline, July 5, 2020, https://deadline.com/2020/07/los-angeles-county-residents-ignore-no-fireworks-order-celebrate-with-massive-display-1202977708.

Index